AI and Drug Development

This important book shines a light on the potential benefits of artificial intelligence (AI) to support advances in drug discovery and development, while also highlighting critical issues around patient confidentiality and ethical practice.

In an era of rapid technological advancement, the book offers a comprehensive assessment of both the challenges and opportunities that AI offers the pharmaceutical sector, explaining how AI and machine learning can support the drug development research process. Illustrated with international case studies that demonstrate how these technologies have already been used to help develop new therapeutic possibilities, it also offers a discussion of ethical concerns around privacy and data protection. By thus taking into account both the technological and ethical issues of AI, the book seeks to present a fair and impartial perspective on the role of AI in further global healthcare.

The book will interest to students and researchers across the Health Science, but particularly in Pharmacy, Pharmacology and related fields, as well as those concerned with AI itself. It will also appeal to practicing pharmacists and pharmacologists working in drug research and development.

Shaik Aminabee, Professor and Head, Department of Pharmacology, Vallabhaneni Venkatadri Institute of Pharmaceutical Sciences, Gudlavalleru, Krishna District, Andhra Pradesh, India.

Atmakuri Lakshmana Rao, Professor and Principal, Vallabhaneni Venkatadri Institute of Pharmaceutical Sciences, Gudlavalleru, Krishna District, Andhra Pradesh, India.

AI and Drug Development

Opportunities, Privacy and Challenges

Shaik Aminabee and
Atmakuri Lakshmana Rao

Routledge
Taylor & Francis Group
LONDON AND NEW YORK

First published 2026
by Routledge
4 Park Square, Milton Park, Abingdon, Oxon OX14 4RN

and by Routledge
605 Third Avenue, New York, NY 10158

Routledge is an imprint of the Taylor & Francis Group, an informa business

British Library Cataloguing-in-Publication Data
A catalogue record for this book is available from the British Library

ISBN: 978-1-041-01737-0 (hbk)
ISBN: 978-1-041-01738-7 (pbk)
ISBN: 978-1-003-61617-7 (ebk)

DOI: 10.4324/9781003616177

Typeset in Times New Roman
by KnowledgeWorks Global Ltd.

Contents

	About the Authors	*vi*
1	Introduction to AI in Drug Discovery	1
2	AI Technologies and Tools in Drug Discovery	23
3	Data Collection and Management for AI in Drug Discovery	48
4	AI-Driven Drug Target Identification	68
5	AI in Drug Design and Optimization	85
6	Preclinical and Clinical Development Using AI	99
7	Regulatory Considerations and Ethical Implications	117
8	Case Studies of AI in Drug Discovery	135
9	Future Trends in AI-Powered Drug Discovery	152
10	Practical Applications and Strategies for Implementation	171
	Index	*187*

About the Authors

Shaik Aminabee received her Bachelor's of Pharmacy from KVSR Siddhartha College of Pharmaceutical Sciences, Vijayawada, in the year 2004 and Master's Degree in Pharmacology from Shri Vishnu College of Pharmacy, Bhimavaram, in the year 2008. She completed a Doctorate Degree from Jawaharlal Nehru Technological University Hyderabad, Kukatpally, in the year 2017. She is presently working as a Professor in the Department of Pharmacology in V. V. Institute of Pharmaceutical Sciences, Gudlavalleru, Andhra Pradesh. She has 15 years of teaching, administrative, and research experience. She was ratified as a Professor from JNTUK, Kakinada, in the year 2024. She has participated in 34 national and international conferences and presented about 29 papers. She acted as a Co-ordinator, Co-convener, and Convener for various international and national conferences. She published 68 articles in reputed journals, out of which 36 are indexed in SCOPUS, 4 in Web of Science, and 1 in PubMed. Gave seven guest lectures. She is a trained nominee for CCSEA, New Delhi, and appointed as a Scientist from Outside the Institute by CCSEA. She acted as the President and Vice-President for the Indian Pharmaceutical Association (IPA) Gudlavalleru Local Branch. She received the Association of Pharmacy Professionals (APP) Best Faculty Award 2017, OPF Oscar Teacher Award of the year 2018, Dr. APJ Abdul Kalam Award for Young Scientist 2019, Young Educator & Scholar Award 2020, and Associate Fellow Award 2021 from AP Akademi of Sciences. She is a Life member of professional societies like IPA, APTI, ISTE, APP, and OPF. She was appointed as a Board Member for Paramedical Sciences at Krishna University, Machilipatnam, in the year 2022. She is currently acting as an Executive Council (EC) Member of JNTUK, appointed by the Government of Andhra Pradesh. She received a 3.5 lakh grant from AICTE under the MODROB Scheme.

Atmakuri Lakshmana Rao received his Bachelor's of Pharmacy from Acharya Nagarjuna University, Nagarjuna Nagar, and Master's Degree in Pharmaceutical Chemistry from Andhra University, Visakhapatnam. He completed the Doctorate Degree from Acharya Nagarjuna University, Nagarjuna Nagar. He has 25 years of Teaching, Administrative, and Research experience. He is presently working as a Principal at V. V. Institute of Pharmaceutical Sciences, Gudlavalleru, Andhra Pradesh. He received several grants from AICTE, PCI, and ISTE. He has guided

13 PhD and 83 MPharm students. He holds eight International and National Patents. He has published six textbooks and three book chapters with prominent publishers. He has participated in 122 national and international conferences. He has presented 43 papers in various international and national conferences. He has organized 60 seminars, conferences, and workshops at national and international levels. He has done extensive research work in the field of Pharmaceutical Sciences and has contributed 430 Research Publications in various reputed International and National Journals. He was invited as a Guest Speaker for 23 seminars and conferences. He has received 40 awards and honors; the prominent among them are Best Oral Presentation Award from Association of Pharmaceutical Teachers of India; Best Principal Award from Council for Skills and Competencies; University Appreciation Award for Senior Principals from Jawaharlal Nehru Technological University Kakinada; Best Oral Presentation Award from Indian Pharmaceutical Association; Pharma Award 2k23 from Andhra Pradesh Pharmacy Council; Best Principal Award from Operant Pharmacy Federation; Prof. M.L. Schroff Pharma Recognition Award from Pharma Lok; Pharmacy Teacher of the Year Award from Pharmacy Teachers Trust; State Best Teacher Award from Government of Andhra Pradesh; Dr. L.V.G. Nargund Research Excellence in Pharmaceutical Chemistry Award from Association of Pharmaceutical Teachers of India; Dr. A.P.J. Abdul Kalam Teacher Excellence Award from Shikshak Kalyan Foundation & AICTE; Best Originality in Research Award from Pharma Middle East Congress, USA; Eminent Pharmacist Award from Operant Pharmacy Federation; Overall First Prize Award from International Medical University, Malaysia; Overall Best Scientific Presentation Award in Indian Pharmaceutical Congress; Nobel Principal of the Year Award from Operant Pharmacy Federation; Principal of the Year Award from Association of Pharmacy Professionals; Meritorious University Best Teacher Award from Jawaharlal Nehru Technological University Kakinada; Best Presentation Award in Indian Pharmaceutical Congress; and Dr. P.D. Sethi Annual Award from Kongposh Publications Pvt. Ltd. He is the editor-in-chief, reviewer, and editorial board member for 143 reputed international and national Journals. He is a life member of professional societies like IPA, APTI, ISTE, ABAP, APP, and OPF.

1 Introduction to AI in Drug Discovery

Introduction: Evolution of Drug Discovery

The need to create medications for expanding health issues has made progress in becoming an essential component of human development. The standard drug discovery approach relies on time-consuming error-based processes which end up being very costly to implement each step of the way. The current research of pharmaceuticals uses artificial intelligence (AI) technology to change the procedures used in discovering and developing pharmaceutical drugs [1].

The Traditional Paradigm of Drug Discovery

The basic methodology of drug development proceeds through consecutive phases starting with target selection and continuing to discover lead chemicals and optimize their properties. Researchers need to identify important biological targets connected to diseases, including proteins and enzymes and genes as their starting point. The identification of lead substances requires scientists to personally test every one of the millions of chemical compounds which bind with the targets. The researchers adjust identified potential lead compounds by modifying their chemical compositions to improve both effectiveness and selectivity and safety aspects [2].

Lab tests and animal trials with scaled drug candidate quantities take place for evaluating both safety and efficiency before preclinical assessments. The medication needs to pass through multiple stages of human clinical trials to earn approval for public distribution [3].

Challenges in the Traditional Drug Discovery Process

The standard drug development method continues to deal with several problems despite recent progress. Most drug candidates fail at the different testing stages which produces both high expenses and prolonged time delays. Many patients are forced to wait several extended years until a medication obtains market approval. Drug development costs create challenges for pharmaceutical companies to obtain financing from discovery through commercial release because these expenses become increasingly hard to sustain over time [4]. Substantial disease understanding

DOI: 10.4324/9781003616177-1

strides have occurred over time, yet medical organizations still struggle to effectively control complex diseases because of the resulting low success rate in developing new treatments.

Artificial Intelligence: A Transformative Solution

Drug discovery uses AI as its revolutionary instrument which has proven better than conventional drug discovery approaches. The combination of AI technology with pharmaceutical research provides scientists with next-level algorithmic processing which makes their work more efficient. AI stimulates drug development through optimized methods that identify targets and optimize leads and design clinical trials [5].

Drug discovery processes reach improved outcomes when AI controls undesired candidates at the initial phases, thus boosting drug development efficiency. The use of AI-based discovery methods creates optimized pathways as well as lowers operational expenses in drug discovery. Through disease simplification processes, cognitive computing systems make it possible for researchers to identify unique therapeutic treatments for different medical conditions. The revolutionary changes to drug discovery procedures speed up research advancement along with providing new solutions to tackle medical problems which currently lack answers [6].

Fundamentals of Artificial Intelligence

Machine Learning

AI contains machine learning as a constituent part allowing computers to discover patterns from data to create predictions and choices automatically. The field comprises three basic learning categories, including supervised learning together with unsupervised learning and reinforcement learning.

The supervised learning process lets algorithms make predictions by processing datasets that combine inputs with their defined output labels. This technique serves as a regular method for handling regression and classification activities [7]. Supervised learning makes possible continuous value prediction through regression but classifies data into distinct groups through classification methods, such as spam detection and disease diagnosis.

The procedure of unsupervised learning functions on unlabeled data to discover regular patterns in unarranged datasets. Clustering is a commonly used method for organizing data points by grouping similar elements into distinct clusters, such as in customer segmentation. The same techniques simplify complex datasets by maintaining important data elements through dimensionality reduction procedures [8].

An agent operating in reinforcement learning participates in environments by taking steps which lead to the receipt of either positive or negative rewards. The learning procedure applies in game-playing AI through AlphaGo and robotics systems which gain optimal strategies through many attempts (Figure 1.1).

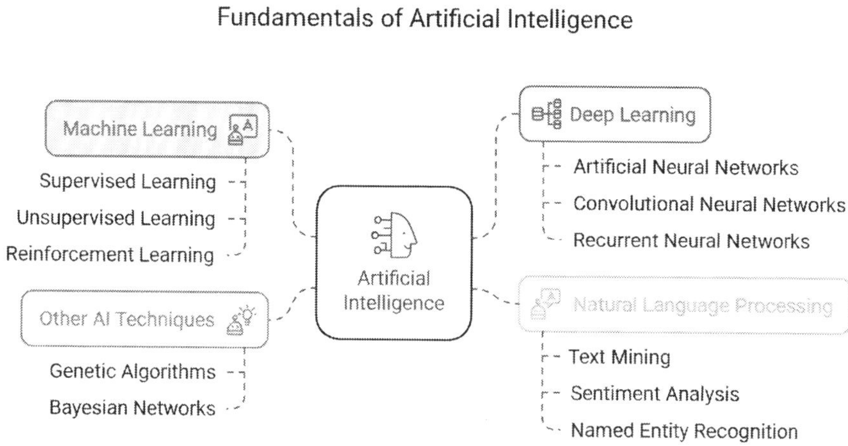

Figure 1.1 Fundamentals of AI

Deep Learning

Artificial neural networks power deep learning which functions as a machine learning specialty that detects complicated data patterns. The networks contain several linked layers that handle information processing in a way that mimics human brain operations [9].

Artificial neural networks form the base for deep learning by using layered connected artificial neurons to understand intricate data structures. Convolutional neural networks (CNNs) function specifically as tools that process image and grid-like data structures. Through their unique architecture, CNNs achieve exceptional results in multiple image-related recognition and detection applications and medical image processing tasks.

Recurrent neural network (RNN) operates as an important deep learning model specially designed to analyze sequential data processing tasks. The RNN serves as a preferred model for natural language processing (NLP) together with speech recognition and time series forecasting because it detects data dependencies across time [10].

Natural Language Processing (NLP)

NLP serves as a field of study which develops systems that let computers process human language while extracting meaning from it and delivering automated responses. The main implementation of NLP technology allows users to extract meaningful information from unlabeled textual data through text mining. Text classification functions as such a method for machine-based sentiment evaluation together with topic extraction. Named entity recognition together with relationship extraction enables the identification of essential textual elements which allows better analysis by structuring information [11].

Sentiment analysis forms a primary NLP research sub-field because it determines emotional text tones which can be either positive or negative or neutral. Scientists apply this technique frequently during the analysis of customer feedback while also utilizing it for social media data collection and market research purposes.

Other AI Techniques

Various AI techniques outside machine learning and deep learning produce solutions that show intelligence for problem-solving. Organisms inspired by principles of natural selection lead to genetic algorithms as one solution. The algorithms base their optimization of complex solutions through crossover and mutation processes primarily for optimization tasks [12].

People utilize Bayesian networks as a substantial AI instrument to show probable variable connections through diagram models. The probabilistic graphical models provide broad applications for decision-making while they assess risks and conduct probabilistic reasoning so users can predict outcomes based on uncertainty modeling.

These AI tools jointly improve the productivity and accuracy along with accelerated data analysis processes across healthcare, finance, and engineering domains [13].

AI Applications in Drug Discovery

Target Identification

Machine learning tools working with AI examine extensive information from RNA sequencing (RNA-seq) datasets to identify genetic expression variations between disease and regular cells. By performing this method, researchers can discover suitable biological drug targets through the detection of particular genes linked to medical conditions. AI functions successfully for advanced studies in cancer treatment along with genetic research [14].

Proteins accomplish their tasks by connecting with other proteins which affects numerous cell functions. AI algorithms detect protein interplay through sequential and structural assessment of protein compounds. The approach stands essential for studying disease origins while helping researchers detect important proteins that contribute to disease development [15].

Lead Discovery

The development of new drugs through traditional methods requires systematic testing of multiple thousands of chemical substances on specific proteins which takes both a great deal of effort and substantial funds. The lead discovery process receives an AI-based enhancement through molecular docking which serves as a virtual screening tool that decides how well drugs attach to their target proteins.

The process of similarity searching allows identification of structurally related compounds that match previously effective medications, while computer-generated scoring functions developed with AI assistance optimize drug affinity measurements and related drug features [16].

AI utilizes de novo drug design technology to produce new drug molecules that researchers did not create before. AI models search and compute various chemical compounds across substantial chemical areas while optimizing drug-like molecule attributes. Ligand-based drug design represents an AI method which detects new chemical compounds through analysis of known drugs or ligands. This method shortens the search for brand-new lead molecules [17].

Lead Optimization

The AI system continues its work on initial lead compounds to both enhance their operational power and minimize adverse reactions. AI algorithms study drug candidate-protein interactions in three dimensions while suggesting modifications of the candidate chemicals that boost recognition strength and selectivity and reduce unwanted effects and drug properties improve drug characteristics like dissolvability and bioavailability and metabolic steadiness [18].

AI helps scientists evaluate how drug candidates absorb into the body and distribute through tissues and metabolize before their elimination. AI predictably analyzes the absorption, distribution, metabolism, excretion, and toxicity (ADMET) properties of drug candidates. Computational prediction of these elements enables researchers to concentrate on compounds with better development outcomes which minimizes wasteful failures during advanced research phases [19].

Preclinical and Clinical Development

Approximately 20 different AI models employ multivariable assessment to forecast preclinical examination outcomes along with clinical trial projections and drug candidate properties, including clinical trial success rate as well as treatment tolerability and best administration protocols [20]. The clinical trial design process achieves improvements through AI through its capabilities to discover the right patient populations as well as define ideal test sizes and research periods and make treatment predictions and biomedical marker detection (Figure 1.2).

The application of AI to trial design lowers expenses while enhancing operational productivity which shortens the time needed for drug approval [21].

Drug Repurposing

The application of AI determines therapeutic uses for drugs that already exist in existing medication libraries [22]. AI extracts valuable information from extensive databases through an analysis of medications alongside illness connections and health system records and scientific journal content to reveal medication side effects as well as extends drug usage into new diseases. The strategic

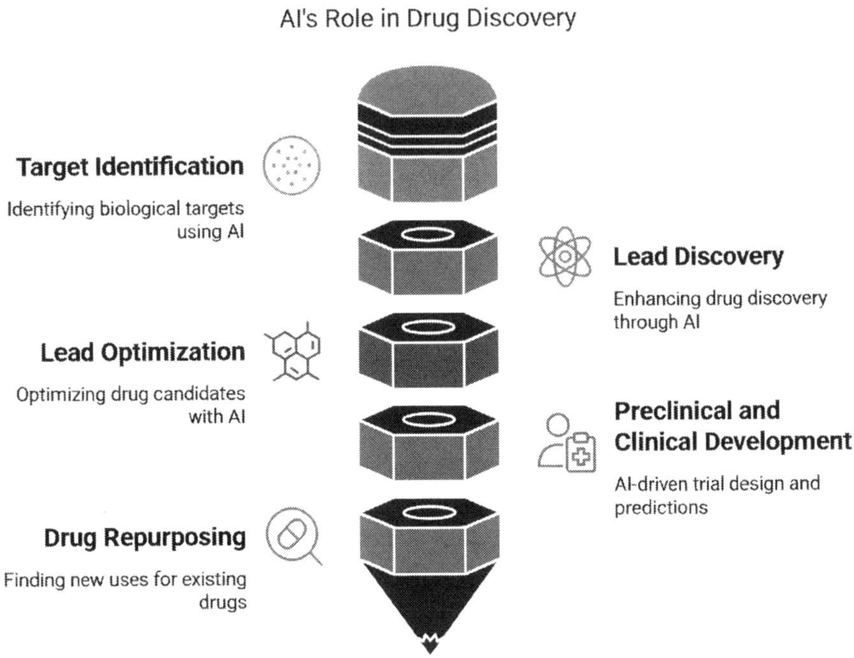

Figure 1.2 Role of AI in Drug Discovery

repurposing of medications proves highly beneficial for scarce diseases since it slashes timeframes and financial expenses needed to produce fresh therapeutic agents [23].

AI-Driven Drug Discovery Pipeline

Integrating AI throughout the Drug Discovery Process

AI will achieve its full impact in drug discovery by becoming perfectly integrated into every aspect of discovery pipelines instead of remaining limited to discrete uses. The necessary approach for success involves a complete ecosystem, including data systems infrastructure alongside AI tool creation and teamwork [24].

Database-driven systems form the basic requirement for drug discovery applications that employ AI. The collection of various datasets comprising experimental gene expression data alongside protein structures as well as chemical libraries and clinical trial data and available publications and text is essential for this process. Clinical testing outcomes and published medical literature with experimental molecular and pharmacological information need to be integrated using standard protocols which enable efficient model development [25]. The AI model needs data quality control systems to ensure accuracy and consistency and data completeness for maintaining model integrity (Figure 1.3).

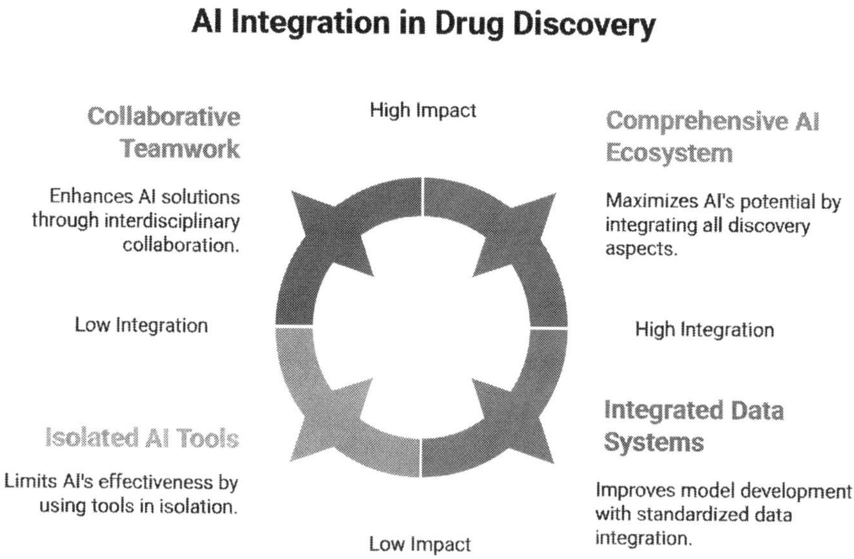

Figure 1.3 AI Integration in Drug Discovery

The creation of AI-driven instruments functions as a key component which supports all stages of drug discovery processes. The association between AI systems enables disease target discovery through their exploration of gene expression patterns and forecasting between proteins. AI tools boost the lead discovery process by carrying out virtual screenings and creating novel drugs while applying ligand-based drug discovery methods [26]. AI-based models provide help to predict ADMET properties and generate medication designs that produce safer and more potent drug substances. The application of AI in clinical research supports data analysis of trial results while enabling scientists to pick optimal patient groups and develop superior treatment plans [27].

The complete utilization of AI in drug discovery demands scientists to work together with data analysts and AI engineers. Organizations need to develop teamwork spaces between scientists and engineers during research to make sure boundaries vanish while debates flourish. The adoption of experimental culture and a learning-by-doing approach will drive better AI solutions in drug discovery [28].

Building an AI-Powered Drug Discovery Platform

An integrated drug discovery system performs as a centralized interface to unite multiple AI technologies and data platforms which guide the whole medication development sequence. A secure data repository functions as a central component in the platform because it understands how to store and structure the enormous quantity of drug discovery data accumulated during processing [29]. Researchers can

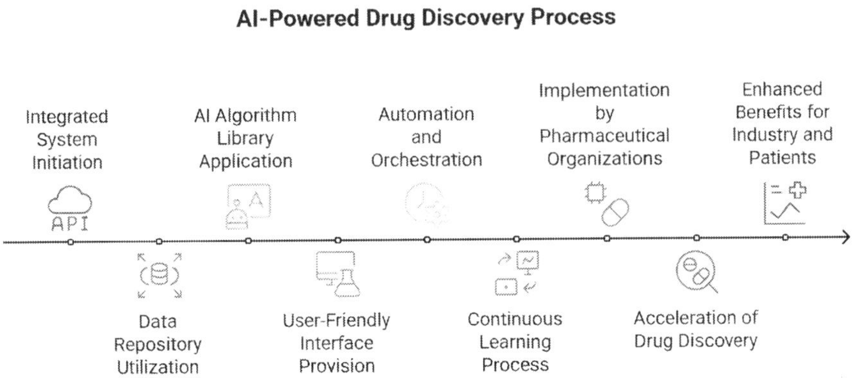

Figure 1.4 Components of AI-Powered Drug Discovery Platform

use the established repository to get critical information efficiently for enhanced analysis and improved decision-making (Figure 1.4).

The essential component includes an AI algorithm library providing both customizable tools and pre-trained AI models which support various application needs. The fundamental capabilities of machine learning models include data classification together with modeling and clustering but deep learning models deliver specialized functions for image processing and NLP and material generation capabilities. Genetic algorithms together with Bayesian networks and reinforcement learning enable the platform to improve its drug discovery workflow optimization according to [30].

The system effectiveness depends on providing researchers a simple and easy-to-use interface which enables anyone from novice to expert to use its features without complexity. The accessible design permits the use of AI technology by pharmaceutical researchers at different research levels [31].

The platform becomes more efficient through automation and orchestration because these features execute background operations that include data preparation tasks together with model training and experimental control. Scientists can boost their drug discovery performance by having AI applications connect to lab protocols which shortens the development time [32].

Learning processes continuously operate as an essential component for systems based on AI. AI models need constant performance analysis along with database and AI technological advancement updates to ensure their effectiveness. System periodic maintenance allows organizations to integrate modern AI techniques which leads to increased model reliability and precision [33].

Pharmaceutical organizations implementing AI-based drug discovery technology obtain multiple key advantages. By using AI technologies, pharmaceutical companies accelerate their medication discovery process, thus shortening the entire development period between target selection and clinical trial commencement. AI-based models generate efficiency which produces cost savings because they decrease experimental failures while implementing resource optimization strategies.

By using AI, pharmaceutical organizations receive two key benefits: the system identifies superior drug possibilities with reduced risk elements. The industry along with patients experiences enhanced benefits from this transformation because it shortens the process to introduce safer and more effective treatments [34].

Success Stories and Case Studies

Real-World Examples of AI-Driven Drug Development

Multiple organizations apply AI technologies effectively to enhance drug development along with enhanced discovery processes. Insilico Medicine shows how AI optimizes drug discovery operations by achieving effective processes in the pharmaceutical industry. Accelerated drug development at the company proceeded at an unprecedented pace after AI revealed a new drug target which led to the creation of a promising candidate drug via shorter methods compared to conventional approaches [35]. The accomplishment showcases how AI capabilities could significantly decrease traditional pharmaceutical drug production expenses and periods (Figure 1.5).

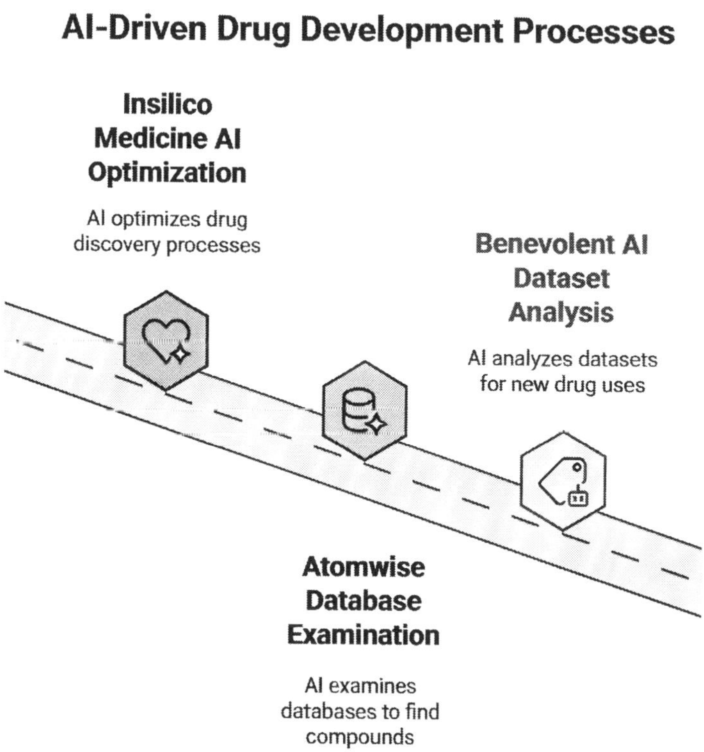

Figure 1.5 AI-Driven Drug Development Process

Atomwise operates as one of the major AI-driven pharmaceutical companies that manages the AtomNet platform through deep learning to enhance drug discovery operations. Through its rapid database examination, AtomNet finds drug candidate compounds accurately. The drug discovery progress for different therapeutic fields has been accelerated through Atomwise's pharmaceutical sector partnerships with multiple companies [36].

Benevolent AI serves as an innovator in AI-powered drug discovery by working to discover new targets along with recasting existing medications for different therapeutic purposes. The company analyzes extensive biomedical datasets of scientific publications and clinical trial results and gene sequences for its AI system to detect fresh disease-drug relationships. The method led to fast discovery of new medical uses for already available drugs in order to accelerate the development of treatments across many medical fields [37].

Lessons Learned and Best Practices

Drug discovery with AI specifically depends on superior quality data resources. The success rate of AI models heavily rests on acquiring well-researched available datasets which follow strict structuring standards. Generating dependable and accurate AI systems depends on building stable methodologies for gathering and organizing and uniting data resources. The achievement of AI drug discovery relies on precise data management to maintain accuracy together with consistency and full datasets [38].

The meaningful application of AI in drug discovery requires domain knowledge about biology, chemistry, and medicine to succeed properly. Expert collaboration between AI specialists with pharmacologists and biochemists and molecular biologists allows relevant data training for AI models to produce scientific results. AI technologies achieve maximum impact through human partnership so they operate as an effective tool for enhancing molecular drug development programs [39].

The required characteristic for AI-driven decisions is the ability to explain their decision-making process clearly and fully. Every precision that AI provides to predictions requires detailed insights regarding the underlying algorithms used for prediction generation. Using Explainable AI (XAI) techniques allows organizations to build model trust because these techniques expose the methods that AI utilizes to make decisions. XAI helps identification of biases along with regulatory compliance through its ability to deliver deep insight about AI algorithms to regulatory authorities who must approve AI-assisted drug discovery [40].

Having robust scalable AI platforms remains essential for complete support of drug discovery operations that benefit from AI. The platforms need to merge perfectly with current research systems to enable smooth teamwork between researchers. These platforms need flexibility because AI technology together with pharmaceutical research will continue to advance through times, therefore requiring integration of emerging approaches and techniques from both fields [41–42].

Ethical Considerations and Societal Impact

Data Privacy and Security

Product development for new drugs depends on gathering substantial sensitive data from patients that involves DNA information and healthcare records and personal information of confidential nature [43]. Creating AI discoveries for drugs depends on valuable patient information which damages their privacy; thus, data security must be an absolute priority. A data breach causes severe issues which include both patient identity theft and financial losses and damage to research institution reputations (Figure 1.6).

Patient information security relies on complete data confidentiality protection as it safeguards private healthcare information from improper usage by individuals who do not have authorization. Organizations performing research need to establish strong privacy defense protocols through advanced encryption and access control systems which deter data burglary [44]. Researchers can preserve study privacy by implementing anonymization tools and de-identification methods when conducting their valuable research work. The scientific research value of patient information remains possible after personal identifiers have been either transformed or eliminated through these protection methods (Table 1.1).

Bias and Fairness in AI Algorithms

AI systems which are trained on biased information will strengthen existing healthcare inequalities since they retain and enlarge existing societal disparities. The performance of AI systems deteriorates drastically when exposed to demographics different from the main training data demographic group due to these discrepancies leading to biased and unjust outcomes. Medical disparities appear due to bias which results in blocked device-based healthcare access and inaccurate predictions of treatment success for diverse patients and uneven medication profiles across groups [45].

The process of reducing bias in AI-based drug discovery requires researchers to build training datasets with complete representation of patient demographics from diverse backgrounds. The collection of data needs to include all demographic groups to avoid result biases [46]. Higher AI fairness levels can be reached through

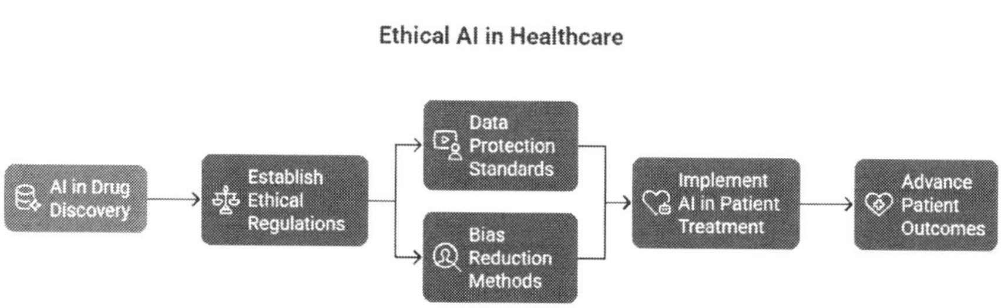

Figure 1.6 Ethical AI in Healthcare

Table 1.1 Data Security Framework for AI in Drug Development

Aspect	*Details*
Sensitive Data in Drug Development	Includes DNA information, healthcare records, and personal confidential data.
Role of AI in Drug Discovery	AI relies on patient data, making privacy and security a critical concern.
Risks of Data Breaches	Patient identity theft Financial losses Damage to research institution reputations
Importance of Data Confidentiality	Ensures private healthcare data is protected from unauthorized access.
Security Measures	Advanced encryption Access control systems Anonymization tools De-identification methods
Preserving Research Value	Research remains valuable by removing personal identifiers while maintaining data integrity.

the use of bias detection systems along with fairness constraints which identify and repair biases that appear in AI decision platforms. AI model evaluation and audit procedures enable researchers to improve datasets and algorithms through new representative datasets that emerge [47].

Access and Equity in AI-Powered Healthcare

AI healthcare solutions require open accessibility for every patient irrespective of their race background together with economic status population distribution or geographical position and cultural heritage. The ability of patients to receive AI-powered treatments remains impeded by three main barriers involving costs alongside limited availability combined with insufficient awareness. These barriers require attention because they affect how AI resources get distributed among various population segments [48].

AI offers promising potential to minimize healthcare gaps because it enhances medical care delivery to underprivileged communities. AI-based healthcare tools developed by organizations must function to uncover health inequality patterns so they can deliver enhanced medical services and custom treatment choices to minority patient populations. Unethical AI utilization can actually increase existing disparities because it will serve patients who access better healthcare more reliably. AI deployment needs proper supervision to stop social inequality reinforcement and establish fair distribution of its advantages [49].

Responsible AI Development and Deployment

Drug discovery through AI requires developers to create systems that maintain transparency while revealing the bases for their decision-making. The capability of AI algorithms to provide prediction methods should be transparent to researchers

Table 1.2 Responsible AI Development and Deployment in Drug Discovery

Key Aspect	*Description*
Transparency and Explainability	AI models must provide interpretable predictions, allowing researchers and healthcare professionals to understand decision-making processes. Explainable AI (XAI) methods help enhance trust and accountability.
Human Oversight	Continuous monitoring by human experts is necessary throughout AI development and deployment to ensure accuracy, safety, and ethical compliance.
Guidelines and Standards	Developers must establish clear guidelines outlining system development protocols, review standards, and intervention measures for responsible AI use.
Performance Evaluation	Regular AI model assessments help identify unintended consequences, security vulnerabilities, and algorithmic biases to maintain reliability.
Ethical Regulations	AI applications in drug discovery and clinical use must comply with ethical guidelines, ensuring patient safety, data protection, and bias minimization.
Regulatory Compliance	Healthcare regulations should set strict criteria for AI deployment, including data security standards, bias mitigation strategies, and responsible implementation in patient care.

and healthcare experts who need this information for making knowledgeable decisions. XAI methods enhance trust because they enable users to interpret AI outcomes, thereby creating accountability of results (Table 1.2).

Monitoring by human experts remains essential from the start to the end of AI program creation and operational implementation. Researchers must develop specific guidelines to clarify system development protocols and review standards as well as intervention procedures for responsible AI application in drug discovery work. Regular monitoring and AI model performance evaluations serve to detect crucial issues that involve unintentional effects and security risks and algorithmic bias detection [50].

Drug discovery together with clinical applications using AI needs proper ethical regulations and procedural standards for their use. Healthcare regulations need to establish specific criteria which define data protection standards together with bias reduction methods and proper practices for implementing AI in patient treatment. The healthcare industry can advance patient results through AI technologies by maintaining ethical practices together with regulatory standards [51].

The Future of AI in Drug Discovery

Emerging Technologies

The field of drug discovery has received considerable advancement due to generative AI technology and its main components, such as Generative Adversarial Networks (GANs) and transformers. The combination of AI technologies produces

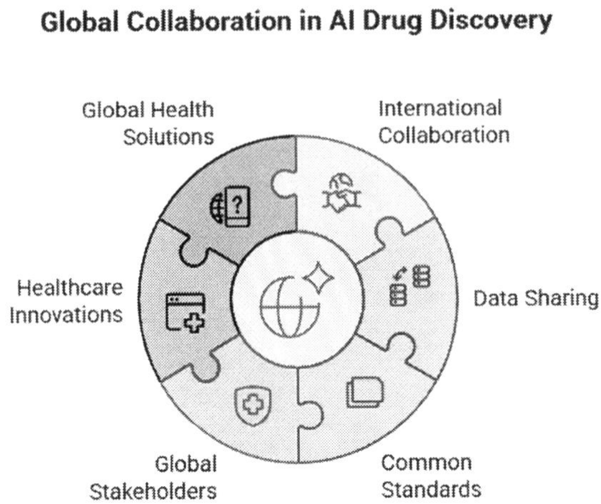

Figure 1.7 Global Collaborations in AI Drug Discovery

new drug molecules via "de novo" drug design processes. Through this method, scientists can access enormous chemical regions which regular drug discovery methods cannot survey [52]. New compounds that fulfill specific targeted properties, including high potency with low toxicity and better bioavailability, can be produced by AI models which boost the search for potential new drug candidates (Figure 1.7).

Quantum computing stands out as one of the most groundbreaking technologies which revolutionizes drug discovery operations. The ability of quantum computers surpasses standard machines since they deliver both highly precise and swift molecular system simulation capabilities [53]. The predictive power of this method directly helps researchers determine protein folding patterns needed for studying drug-protein behavior. Higher accuracy emerges from quantum computing when running drug-target interaction simulations and this leads to more precise drug response analyses. A quick exploration method for extensive chemical domains shortens drug development cycles, thus shifting pharmaceutical timelines for new drug releases [54].

Challenges and Opportunities

The main barrier to AI-driven drug discovery resides in obtaining high-quality varied data that has been properly curated. The success of AI predictions depends heavily on extensive datasets so scientists struggle with insufficient data for accurate and transferable forecasting. Multiple organizations should work together to combine data points from clinical trials and electronic health records and public databases to improve both data quality and accessibility [55].

The issues of interpretability together with explainability stand as essential matters for consideration. The deep learning models operate like black boxes since they produce decisions without providing easy understanding of their internal processes. The inability to see how AI systems work causes problems for trust in drug discovery applications and complicates safety standard approval procedures. XAI techniques need development to generate interpretive and transparent models that show how predictions occur [56].

Ethical considerations represent a main concern in drug discovery systems. Drug discovery AI applications need to solve problems which include protected data and unbiased algorithm creation and fair medical treatment availability to all groups. Public trust depends on maintaining ethical AI practices, while equitable distribution of AI-driven healthcare solutions requires these ethical practices to remain in place [57].

Obstacles related to regulatory requirements function as major barriers during this process. Winning regulatory approval for AI-based therapeutics requires organizations to move through complicated rules that become labor-intensive and complex during the process. The development of AI-based drug products requires clear comprehensive regulatory guidelines which must create standardized implementation procedures [58].

Technology challenges do not prevent AI from delivering extensive potential prospects to drug discovery efforts. AI detection systems speed up pharmaceutical research through better target finding capabilities and optimize clinical trial procedures while minimizing the total time needed to deliver new medical treatments to healthcare providers. The analysis capacity of AI allows it to process large data collections which results in better medicines with reduced side effects [59].

The ability of AI programs enables medical research that develops new treatments for challenging diseases which include both rare health problems and disorders affecting the nervous system. Modern developments in AI have led to personalized medicine treatments which provide individualized treatment plans based on patient characteristics for optimized drug outcomes [60].

The Role of Collaboration and Partnerships

A combination of stakeholder cooperation extending across different industries and disciplines produces the highest effectiveness for AI-based drug discovery. AI-based drug discovery advancements are strongly supported by the collaborations that exist between pharmaceutical companies together with both academic institutions and technology firms. Through partnerships, pharmaceutical organizations gain access to academic research knowledge along with innovative technological solutions for their drug development system [61].

The accomplishment of AI-based drug discovery relies on the establishment of public-private partnerships. Organizations, such as governments and regulatory bodies, should cooperate with private organizations to exchange vital information while sharing valuable practice examples [62]. Public agencies help develop AI research through financial support for infrastructure building and establishment of healthcare AI implementation standards [63].

A collaborative approach between worldwide institutions remains vital because it will make AI-powered drug discovery accessible to healthcare systems worldwide [64]. The sharing of data with worldwide partners through international collaborations allows organizations to exchange information and adopt common standards for best practices throughout international borders. Global stakeholders working together can improve AI-driven healthcare innovations access as well as find solutions to worldwide health problems with increased effectiveness [65].

Conclusion: A New Era of Drug Discovery

The Transformative Potential of AI

AI technologies will transform pharmaceutical research because they speed up the entire drug creation process at reduced expenses. The development of new drugs becomes faster because traditional drug methods are expensive and time-consuming, yet modern AI technology simplifies compound screening alongside data analysis [66]. The streamlined approach enabled by AI brings forth lifesaving treatment options to patients which results in superior healthcare results.

AI offers drug development its most valuable advantage by enhancing therapeutic results. The effectiveness of AI-driven therapies increases because they reduce adverse side effects during development [67]. The analysis of extensive datasets through AI allows pharmaceutical scientists to create drugs that achieve better results combined with specific modes of action and improved secure features. Better patient care outcomes result from these improvements which bring about better life quality for patients.

AI technology functions as a vital platform to resolve healthcare demands that have yet to receive medical solutions. Numerous medical conditions, including rare diseases and neurodegenerative disorders together with infectious diseases, have no available effective treatments at present. The combination of modern AI tools with drug development enables researchers to detect new target areas while creating new therapeutic methods which speed up discoveries of difficult disease medications [68]. Medical progress through this technology creates possibilities of getting treatment to patients who need it but have no current therapeutic options available.

AI-based drug discovery brings personalized medicine forward as a major transformational aspect. Through AI-developed systems, scientists can create treatments that specifically address the distinct characteristics found in individual patients, including their genes and their medical histories and their personal lifestyles [69]. AI analyzes different variables to forecast therapeutic results and enhance drug dosages in combination with reduced risks of adverse drug reactions. This individualized strategy delivers patients their most efficient treatment options which additionally minimize their chances of adverse side effects [70].

AI makes drug development more successful because it enhances predictive abilities. AI-driven predictive models assist medical researchers to identify successful drug candidates with higher efficiency, thus decreasing the occurrence of unsuccessful clinical trials. The optimized approach enhances treatment availability by reducing time and costs and expedites new effective treatments access for patients [71].

Future Directions and Research Priorities

Progress in AI-driven drug discovery depends on steady improvements of modern AI technological advancements. Science investigators need to work on boosting AI capability development specifically in generative AI and reinforcement learning and XAI methods. AI scientific progress will generate new possibilities for pharmaceutical development by producing innovative drug molecules and better results for targeted treatment [72]. The application of quantum computing technologies shows great potential to enhance drug discovery capabilities by providing superior molecular interaction simulations while speeding up the drug discovery process for better therapeutic results.

Data-related problems represent a fundamental prerequisite for progressing AI applications within drug discovery projects. An effective training of AI models requires clinical data that maintains high-quality standards and displays diversity within proper annotation standards. Researchers should construct techniques to both maintain data reliability and accessibility of these datasets and resolve privacy and security issues with the information. The development of AI-driven drug discovery requires complete integration and processing of information collected from clinical trials with electronic health records and genomic databases [73].

Corporate healthcare depends on creating AI systems that demonstrate both strength and moral integrity. Software programs built for healthcare applications require engineers to develop decision systems which demonstrate reliability and transparency alongside fairness. Organizations need to establish methods that limit AI algorithm biases while designing decision-explaining systems which reveal the reasoning behind their decisions. In order to benefit all patients, the healthcare system prioritizes three key ethical elements, including patient data security together with program transparency and equal treatment accessibility for AI-controlled medical treatments [74].

AI-powered drug discovery needs the critical support of both collaborations between stakeholders and partnership development. Research and development success within this domain mandates close relationships between practitioners of different professional specialties, including data scientists along with clinicians and researchers. Academic institutions along with pharmaceutical firms and government agencies establish productive public-private partnerships to exchange knowledge and distribute resources besides creating uniform best practices standards. AI-driven drug discovery technologies require such partnerships to achieve successful implementation according to [75].

The future of AI drug discovery depends heavily on spending money on education together with training programs. Professionals at different levels as well as researchers need appropriate training in AI and both data science and computational biology. AI-related instructional elements should become part of educational programs to teach the future generation of scientists together with healthcare professionals about the expanding importance of AI in medical settings. The scientific community will achieve maximum AI drug discovery and healthcare benefits through proper education of fundamental skills and knowledge for individuals.

References

1. Mullard, A. (2020). The drug developer's guide to the galaxy. *Nature Reviews Drug Discovery*, *19*(11), 739–741.
2. Imming, P., Sinning, C., & Meyer, A. (2006). Drugs, their targets, and the nature and number of drug targets. *Nature Reviews Drug Discovery*, *5*(10), 821–834.
3. Santos, R., Ursu, O., Gaulton, A., Bento, A. P., Donadi, R. S., Bologa, C. G., & Overington, J. P. (2017). A comprehensive map of molecular drug targets. *Nature Reviews Drug Discovery*, *16*(1), 19–34.
4. Paul, S. M., Mytelka, D. S., Dunwiddie, C. T., Persinger, C. C., Munos, B. H., Lindborg, S. R., & Schacht, A. L. (2010). How to improve R&D productivity: The pharmaceutical industry's grand challenge. *Nature Reviews Drug Discovery*, *9*(3), 203–214.
5. DiMasi, J. A., Grabowski, H. G., & Hansen, R. W. (2016). Innovation in the pharmaceutical industry: New estimates of R&D costs. *Journal of Health Economics*, *47*, 20–33.
6. Aminabee, S. K., Prabhakar, M. C., Prasad, R. G. S. V., & Lakshmana Rao, A. (2011). Screening the pharmacological activity of cerium oxide nanoparticles in-vitro. *Biomedical and Pharmacology Journal*, *4*(2), 287–289.
7. Schmidhuber, J. (2015). Deep learning in neural networks: An overview. *Neural Networks*, *61*, 85–117.
8. LeCun, Y., Bengio, Y., & Hinton, G. (2015). Deep learning. *Nature*, *521*(7553), 436–444.
9. Chen, H., Engkvist, O., Wang, Y., Olivecrona, M., & Blaschke, T. (2018). The rise of deep learning in drug discovery. *Drug Discovery Today*, *23*(6), 1241–1250.
10. Walters, W. P., Barzilay, R., & Davies, J. W. (2021). Applications of deep learning in drug discovery. *Current Opinion in Chemical Biology*, *65*, 105–113.
11. Schneider, G. (2018). Automating drug discovery. *Nature Reviews Drug Discovery*, *17*(2), 97–113.
12. Zhavoronkov, A., Ivanenkov, Y. A., Aliper, A., Veselov, M. S., Aladinskiy, V. A., Aladinskaya, A. V., …, & Aspuru-Guzik, A. (2019). Artificial intelligence in drug discovery. *Nature Biotechnology*, *37*(4), 360–370.
13. Aminabee, S. K., Lakshmana Rao, A., Sowmya, K., Nymisha, D., Kusuma Naga Lakshmi, K., Manikanta, K. V. N. S., & Praveen Kumar, P. (2019). Evaluation of analgesic activity of *Ficus palmata. Iranian Journal of Pharmaceutical Sciences*, *15*(3), 47–60.
14. Gawehn, E., Hiss, J. A., & Schneider, G. (2016). Deep learning in drug discovery. *Molecular Informatics*, *35*(1), 3–14.
15. Patel, L., Shukla, T., Huang, X., Ussery, D. W., & Wang, S. (2020). Machine learning methods in drug discovery. *Molecules*, *25*(22), 5277.
16. Zhavoronkov, A. (2018). Deep learning for drug discovery: A guide to the future. *Drug Discovery Today*, *23*(11), 2107–2115.
17. Vamathevan, J., Clark, D., Czodrowski, P., Dunham, I., Ferran, E., Lee, G., …, & Zhao, S. (2019). Applications of machine learning in drug discovery and development. *Nature Reviews Drug Discovery*, *18*(6), 463–477.
18. Aminabee, S. K., & Lakshmana Rao, A. (2022). Clinical trials status and approaches of COVID-19 vaccines developed globally: The recent updates. *Pharma Times*, *54*(3), 7–14.

19. Chan, H. C. S., Shan, H., Dahoun, T., Vogel, H., & Yuan, S. (2019). Advancing drug discovery via artificial intelligence. *Trends in Pharmacological Sciences*, *40*(8), 592–604.
20. Zeng, X., Song, X., Ma, T., Pan, X., Zhou, Y., Hou, Y., & Yang, L. (2022). AI4Drug: Repurposing FDA-approved drugs against COVID-19 through machine learning and drug–target interaction modeling. *Briefings in Bioinformatics*, *23*(1), bbab460.
21. Aminabee, S. K., Lakshmana Rao, A., & Chinna Eswaraiah, M. (2020). In-vivo antioxidant activity of different fractions of *Indigofera barberi* against paracetamol-induced toxicity in rats. *Turkish Journal of Pharmaceutical Sciences*, *17*(2), 136–140.
22. Bung, N., Krishnan, S. R., Bulusu, G., Roy, A., Amato, C., & Kanevsky, M. (2021). De novo design of new chemical entities (NCEs) for SARS-CoV-2 using artificial intelligence. *Future Medicinal Chemistry*, *13*(6), 575–585.
23. Wang, Y., Zhang, S., Li, F., Zhou, Y., Zhang, Y., Wang, Z., & Chen, Y. (2020). Therapeutic target database 2020: Enriched resource for facilitating research and early development of targeted therapeutics. *Nucleic Acids Research*, *48*(D1), D1031–D1041.
24. Wishart, D. S., Knox, C., Guo, A. C., Cheng, D., Shrivastava, S., Tzur, D., & Woolsey, J. (2008). DrugBank: A knowledgebase for drugs, drug actions and drug targets. *Nucleic Acids Research*, *36*(suppl_1), D901–D906.
25. Gaulton, A., Hersey, A., Nowotka, M., Bento, A. P., Chambers, J., Mendez, D., & Leach, A. R. (2017). The ChEMBL database in 2017. *Nucleic Acids Research*, *45*(D1), D945–D954.
26. Prasanth, D. S. N. B. K., Aminabee, S. K., Lakshmana Rao, A., Teja, N., Bhargavi, K., Monika, C., Pujitha, B., Sandhya, T., Lalitha, A., & Siva Prasad, P. (2020). Anthelmintic activity of *Mansoa alliacea* against *Pheretima posthuma*: In-vitro and in-silico approach. *Thai Journal of Pharmaceutical Sciences*, *4*(3), 186–196.
27. Irwin, J. J., & Shoichet, B. K. (2005). ZINC – a free database of commercially available compounds for virtual screening. *Journal of Chemical Information and Modeling*, *45*(1), 177–182.
28. Berman, H. M., Westbrook, J., Feng, Z., Gilliland, G., Bhat, T. N., Weissig, H., & Bourne, P. E. (2000). The protein data bank. *Nucleic Acids Research*, *28*(1), 235–242.
29. Szklarczyk, D., Gable, A. L., Lyon, D., Junge, A., Wyder, S., Huerta-Cepas, J., & Morris, J. H. (2019). STRING v11: Protein–protein association networks with increased coverage, supporting functional discovery in genome-wide experimental datasets. *Nucleic Acids Research*, *47*(D1), D607–D613.
30. Wishart, D. S., Feunang, Y. D., Guo, A. C., Lo, E. J., Marcu, A., Grant, J. R., & Wilson, M. (2018). DrugBank 5.0: A major update to the DrugBank database for 2018. *Nucleic Acids Research*, *46*(D1), D1074–D1082.
31. Chen, B., Ding, Y., & Wild, D. J. (2012). Assessing drug target association using semantic linked data. *PLoS Computational Biology*, *8*(7), e1002574.
32. Oprea, T. I., Bologa, C. G., Brunak, S., Campbell, A., Gan, G. N., Gaulton, A., & Sklar, L. A. (2018). Unexplored therapeutic opportunities in the human genome. *Nature Reviews Drug Discovery*, *17*(5), 377.
33. Kim, S., Chen, J., Cheng, T., Gindulyte, A., He, J., He, S., …, & Bolton, E. E. (2019). PubChem 2019 update: Improved access to chemical data. *Nucleic Acids Research*, *47*(D1), D1102–D1109.
34. Prasanth, D. S. N. B. K., Aminabee, S. K., Lakshmana Rao, A., Guntupalli, C., Reddy, A. R., Kulandaivelu, U., Rao, S. N. K., & Rajeshwari, P. (2021). Inhibitory effects of *Mansoa alliacea* in Freund's adjuvant arthritis on inflammatory markers and its confirmation by in-silico strategy. *Thai Journal of Pharmaceutical Sciences*, *45*(6), 532–544.
35. Goh, G. B., Siegel, C., Vishnu, A., Hodas, N. O., & Baker, N. (2017). Chemception: A deep neural network with minimal chemistry knowledge matches the performance of expert-developed QSAR/QSPR models. *ACS Central Science*, *3*(8), 852–859.

36. Wu, Z., Ramsundar, B., Feinberg, E. N., Gomes, J., Geniesse, C., Pappu, A. S., & Pande, V. (2018). MoleculeNet: A benchmark for molecular machine learning. *Chemical Science*, *9*(2), 513–530.
37. Rogers, D., & Hahn, M. (2010). Extended-connectivity fingerprints. *Journal of Chemical Information and Modeling*, *50*(5), 742–754.
38. Segler, M. H. S., Preuss, M., & Waller, M. P. (2018). Planning chemical syntheses with deep neural networks and symbolic AI. *Nature*, *555*(7698), 604–610.
39. Ravi Shankar, K., Aminabee, S. K., Chenchu Lakshmi, K. N. V., Ramana Reddy, G., Reehana, S. K., Vineetha, T., Almaas Sultana, S. K., Basha, S. K., Mokesh Sai, K., Bhagavan, J., & Dinesh Kumar, C. (2023). Effect of various sustained release polymers on floating tablets of carvedilol phosphate - A comparative study. *International Journal of Applied Pharmaceutics*, *15*(6), 125–131.
40. Schwaller, P., Petraglia, R., Zullo, V., Nair, V. H., Haeuselmann, R. A., Pisoni, R., & Laino, T. (2021). Predicting retrosynthetic pathways using transformer-based models and a hyper-graph exploration strategy. *Chemical Science*, *12*(9), 3339–3349.
41. Elton, D. C., Boukouvalas, Z., Fuge, M. D., & Chung, P. W. (2019). Deep learning for molecular design - A review of the state of the art. *Molecular Systems Design & Engineering*, *4*(4), 828–849.
42. Aminabee, S. K., Santhi Krupa, D., Hanumanth Rao, K., Sirisha, V., Anitha Kumari, V., Nagasen, D., Sujiya, B., & Leelavati, T. S. (2023). Pharmacoeconomic analysis of biologic vs. biosimilar therapies in rheumatoid arthritis. *International Journal of Chemical and Biochemical Sciences*, *24*(4), 395–400.
43. Stokes, J. M., Yang, K., Swanson, K., Jin, W., Cubillos-Ruiz, A., Donghia, N. M., & Collins, J. J. (2020). A deep learning approach to antibiotic discovery. *Cell*, *180*(4), 688–702.e13.
44. Zhavoronkov, A., Ivanenkov, Y. A., Aliper, A., Veselov, M. S., Aladinskiy, V. A., Aladinskaya, A. V., & Zholus, A. (2019). Deep learning enables rapid identification of potent DDR1 kinase inhibitors. *Nature Biotechnology*, *37*(9), 1038–1040.
45. Segler, M. H. S., & Waller, M. P. (2017). Neural-symbolic machine learning for retrosynthesis and reaction prediction. *Chemistry–A European Journal*, *23*(25), 5966–5971.
46. Schneider, G., & Clark, D. E. (2019). Automated de novo drug design: Are we nearly there yet? *Angewandte Chemie International Edition*, *58*(32), 10792–10803.
47. Leelavati, T. S., Madhavi, S., & Aminabee, S. (2025). Fostering ethical decision-making skills in pharmaceutical education: Vital for future pharmacists. *Indian Journal of Pharmaceutical Education and Research*, *59*(2), 433–440.
48. Kadurin, A., Nikolenko, S., Khrabrov, K., Aliper, A., & Zhavoronkov, A. (2017). druGAN: An advanced generative adversarial autoencoder model for de novo generation of new molecules with desired molecular properties in silico. *Molecular Pharmaceutics*, *14*(9), 3098–3104.
49. Leelavati, T. S., Madhavi, S., Kamal, G., Raju, P. V. M., Susmitha, K., Vinod, M., & Aminabee, S. K. (2023). Revolutionizing healthcare delivery: Telemedicine's influence on access and patient satisfaction. *International Journal of Chemical and Biochemical Sciences*, *24*(5), 106–115.
50. Blaschke, T., Olivecrona, M., Engkvist, O., Bajorath, J., & Chen, H. (2018). Application of generative autoencoder in de novo molecular design. *Molecular Informatics*, *37*(1–2), 1700123.
51. Gao, W., & Coley, C. W. (2020). The synthesizability of molecules proposed by generative models. *Journal of Chemical Information and Modeling*, *60*(12), 5714–5723.
52. Winter, R., Montanari, F., Noé, F., & Clevert, D. A. (2019). Learning continuous and data-driven molecular descriptors by translating equivalent chemical representations. *Chemical Science*, *10*(6), 1692–1701.
53. Brown, N., Fiscato, M., Segler, M. H. S., & Vaucher, A. C. (2019). GuacaMol: Benchmarking models for de novo molecular design. *Journal of Chemical Information and Modeling*, *59*(3), 1096–1108.

54. Gómez-Bombarelli, R., Wei, J. N., Duvenaud, D., Hernández-Lobato, J. M., Sánchez-Lengeling, B., Sheberla, D., & Aspuru-Guzik, A. (2018). Automatic chemical design using a data-driven continuous representation of molecules. *ACS Central Science*, *4*(2), 268–276.
55. Aminabee, S. K., Devi Mallika, K., & Lakshmana Rao, A. (2023). Natural resources in management and treatment of diseases: A review. *Pharma Times*, *55*(11), 7–10.
56. Olivecrona, M., Blaschke, T., Engkvist, O., & Chen, H. (2017). Molecular de novo design through deep reinforcement learning. *Journal of Cheminformatics*, *9*, 48.
57. Popova, M., Isayev, O., & Tropsha, A. (2018). Deep reinforcement learning for de novo drug design. *Science Advances*, *4*(7), eaap7885.
58. Jha, S., Majumdar, A., & Saha, S. (2022). Role of artificial intelligence in drug discovery and development. *International Journal of Molecular Sciences*, *23*(8), 4445.
59. Ganga Raju, K., Varaprasad Goud, P., Parween, S., Ramarao, M., Leelavati, T. S., Madhavi, S., & Aminabee, S. (2024). Economic analysis of pharmacological interventions for substance use disorders: Cost-effectiveness and market dynamics. *Journal of Drug and Alcohol Research*, *13*(7), 1–4.
60. Wang, Y., Zeng, J., & Cui, Y. (2021). Drug discovery with explainable deep learning. *Current Opinion in Pharmacology*, *57*, 124–130.
61. Wu, C., Zhu, Z., Wang, Y., Xia, J., & Zeng, J. (2021). Graph neural networks in computer-aided drug design: Method and application. *Chemical Reviews*, *121*(16), 11238–11288.
62. Gilmer, J., Schoenholz, S. S., Riley, P. F., Vinyals, O., & Dahl, G. E. (2017). Neural message passing for quantum chemistry. *Proceedings of the 34th International Conference on Machine Learning*, *70*, 1263–1272.
63. Aminabee, S. K., & Lakshmana Rao, A. (2024). Computational identification of selected bioactive compounds from *Cedrus deodara* as inhibitors against SARS-CoV-2 main protease: A pharmacoinformatics study. *Indian Drugs*, *61*(2), 78–91.
64. Mendez-Lucio, O., Baillif, B., Clevert, D. A., Rouquie, D., & Wichard, J. (2020). De novo generation of hit-like molecules from gene expression signatures using artificial intelligence. *Nature Communications*, *11*(1), 10.
65. Kim, H., Na, H., Song, M., & Yoon, S. (2021). A deep learning model for molecular structure prediction from MS/MS spectra. *Nature Communications*, *12*, 5255.
66. Ragoza, M., Hochuli, J., Idrobo, E., Sunseri, J., & Koes, D. R. (2017). Protein–ligand scoring with convolutional neural networks. *Journal of Chemical Information and Modeling*, *57*(4), 942–957.
67. Stepniewska-Dziubinska, M. M., Zielenkiewicz, P., & Siedlecki, P. (2018). Development and evaluation of a deep learning model for protein–ligand binding affinity prediction. *Bioinformatics*, *34*(21), 3666–3674.
68. Karimi, M., Wu, D., Wang, Z., & Shen, Y. (2019). DeepAffinity: Interpretable deep learning of compound protein affinity through unified recurrent and convolutional neural networks. *Bioinformatics*, *35*(18), 3329–3338.
69. Aminabee, S. K., Ravi Shankar, K., Chenchu Lakshmi, K. N. V., Saritha, K., Kavya, R., Chaitanya Babu, K., & Santhi Krupa, D. (2024). Influence of Allium sativum on the hypoglycaemic activity of gliclazide in normal rats: A possible approach to herb-drug interaction. *Biomedical and Pharmacology Journal*, *17*(1), 377–382.
70. He, T., Heidemeyer, M., Ban, F., Cherkasov, A., & Ester, M. (2017). SimBoost: A read-across approach for predicting drug–target binding affinities using gradient boosting machines. *Journal of Cheminformatics*, *9*, 24. https://doi.org/10.1186/s13321-017-0209-z
71. Ozturk, H., Ozgur, A., & Ozkirimli, E. (2018). Deep DTA: Deep drug–target binding affinity prediction. *Bioinformatics*, *34*(17), i821–i829.
72. Lee, I., Keum, J., & Nam, H. (2019). DeepConv-DTI: Prediction of drug–target interactions via deep learning with convolution on protein sequences. *PLoS Computational Biology*, *15*(6), e1007129.

73. Ravi Shankar, K., Aminabee, S. K., Ramana, G., Chenchu Lakshmi, K. N. V., & Indusree, G. (2024). Formulation and evaluation of propranolol hydrochloride floating tablets by 32 factorial design. *International Journal of Drug Delivery Technology*, *14*(4), 2060–2067.
74. Tang, J., Szwajda, A., Shakyawar, S., Xu, T., Hintsanen, P., Wennerberg, K., & Aittokallio, T. (2014). Making sense of large-scale kinase inhibitor bioactivity data sets: A comparative and integrative analysis. *Journal of Chemical Information and Modeling*, *54*(3), 735–743.
75. Keiser, M. J., Setola, V., Irwin, J. J., Laggner, C., Abbas, A. I., Hufeisen, S. J., & Roth, B. L. (2009). Predicting new molecular targets for known drugs. *Nature*, *462*(7270), 175–181.

2 AI Technologies and Tools in Drug Discovery

Introduction

Artificial Intelligence (AI) functions as a revolutionary power that modifies traditional pharmaceutical operations related to drug discovery and development. Drug discovery approaches that used traditional methods require numerous resources and extended times due to their challenging nature and high costs as it can take more than 10 years to produce new medicines. Drugs are optimized through each phase of development by AI technology and its combination of machine learning (ML) and deep learning (DL) methods and big data analysis [1]. Modern technologies process and predict data and execute automated workflows which shorten both drug discovery processes and resources needed to verify new drug possibilities. AI makes it possible to discover fresh drug targets and boost drug renovation initiatives and helps doctors organize clinical trial participants more effectively. The combination of AI technologies within drug discovery practices enables pharmaceutical organizations to develop new therapeutic interventions faster with decreased expense and higher successful results.

Evolution of AI in Pharmaceutical Sciences

AI technology has progressed in pharmaceutical sciences through stages which started from simple computational modeling before reaching advanced AI-based drug discovery platforms. Drug discovery projects from the past depended on computational chemistry together with structure-activity relationship (SAR) models for making molecular compound behavior predictions [2]. The employed methods demonstrated restricted capabilities when dealing with extensive biological systems as well as large-scale datasets. ML and DL elements of AI have changed data analysis systems by allowing very large dataset processing together with predictive analytics and automated decision systems.

AI platforms examine big genomic and proteomic and metabolomic datasets to find drug targets and forecast molecular behavior with excellent precision. AI tools that run natural language processing (NLP) algorithms enable researchers to extract important scientific information from published literature and clinical reports and patents which speeds up research productivity in drug discovery [3]. AI technologies flow through various elements of pharmaceutical research which brings speed

DOI: 10.4324/9781003616177-2

and data-based performance to drug development protocols and clinical trials and preclinical assessment stages and leads and target discovery operations.

Role of AI in Accelerating Drug Development Pipelines

The drug development process experiences acceleration through AI technology which optimizes various important steps starting from target identification until clinical trials. AI programs search through extensive biological data collections to determine disease-related genes and proteins and biological pathways which leads to better therapeutic target selection. Virtual screening methods powered by AI allow scientists to speed up chemical compound assessments for precise prediction of their ability to bind targets and their pharmaceutical effects [4]. The process requires fewer time-consuming and expensive experimental testing methods. AI discovers novel therapeutic uses for available medications by making factual-based discoveries.

The absorption distribution metabolism excretion and toxicity (ADMET) properties of drug candidates can be forecasted using AI-based in silico models during preclinical stages to eliminate compounds with unfavorable attributes in the beginning of development. AI optimizes clinical trials through better patient recruitment strategies and it helps designers build improved trial plans while enabling real-time patient response monitoring. AI predictive analytics system selects appropriate clinical trial subjects through the analysis of patient biomarkers combined with genetic information leading to better trial performance [5]. AI helps regulatory organizations achieve automated data evaluation in their drug approval evaluation while also performing post-market monitoring procedures. Pharmaceutical corporations that embed AI throughout all drug developing stages achieve faster new drug deployment with reduced research time and less development failures.

Impact of AI on Cost Reduction and Success Rates in Drug Discovery

The implementation of AI results in cheaper drug discovery operations together with heightened success rates. Billions of dollars stand as typical expenses during drug discovery operations because preclinical and clinical trial failure rates remain high. The implementation of AI predictive models works to decrease financial burdens because they enhance early stage forecasting precision, thus minimizing late stage candidate failure rates. The application of ML technologies examines previous drug development records to detect successful project markers, which helps researchers find better pharmaceutical substances [6]. The data-driven method helps organizations prevent investment in compounds that show low effectiveness and adverse safety characteristics.

AI demonstrates major cost reduction capabilities through its drug reassignment abilities. Large biomedical databases along with electronic health records (EHRs) and clinical trial data get processed by AI algorithms which produce identification results of drugs eligible for new therapeutic applications. The use of already evaluated drugs for new indications decreases both development cost and time to market since these validated medications have met safety standards [7]. The use of AI brings improvement to resource management by enhancing laboratory procedures while cutting down the need for excessive laboratory work and improving

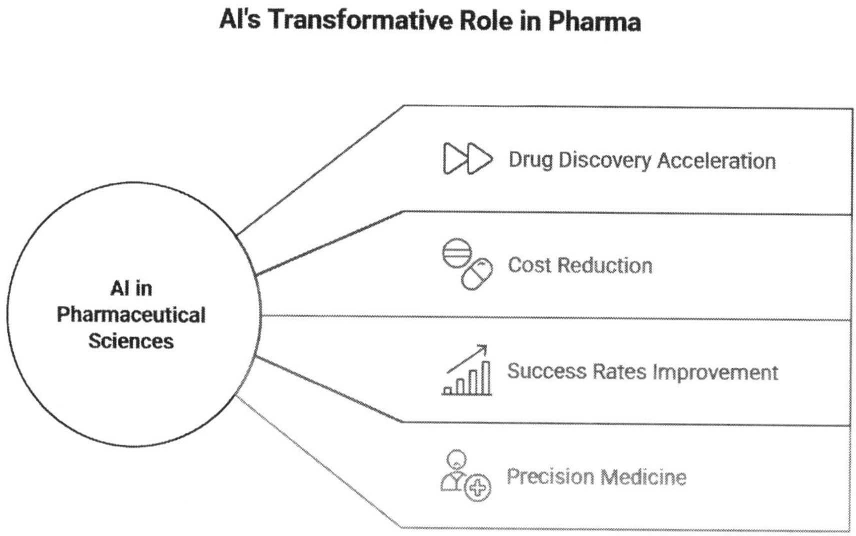

Figure 2.1 AIs Transformative Role in Pharma

production operations. Operations become more efficient through automated functions of chemical synthesis together with high-throughput screening (HTS) and quality control procedures while also decreasing labor expenses (Figure 2.1).

AI-based precision medicine strategies elevate treatment outcomes when healthcare providers develop personalized medicine plans for patients through their disease-related molecular data. Through its ability to match patients with optimal therapies while minimizing unfavorable drug reactions, AI both enhances medical care results and lowers health system expenses [8]. AI demonstrates immense value in pharmaceutical sciences by reducing costs while maximizing both the success rates of new discoveries and development outcomes in pharmaceutical technologies.

AI Technologies Transforming Drug Discovery

AI brought a transformative change to drug discovery through its ability to perform high throughout data analysis while making decisions based on data and achieve precise compound optimization in therapeutic drug development. The implementation of AI systems helps drug developers complete all steps in the development process starting from target selection moving through trial planning and shortening both development duration and expense needed for releasing new medicines. Through the application of ML and DL as well as generative AI and NLP and reinforcement learning (RL), pharmaceutical researchers and companies can now conduct more efficient and effective exploration of new drug candidates and biological interaction predictions and molecular property optimization [9]. New technologies under development have transformed how drugs are discovered because they introduce systematic processes that enable scalable operations for addressing difficult diseases (Table 2.1).

Table 2.1 AI Technologies Transforming Drug Discovery

AI Technology	*Description*	*Examples*	*Key Benefits*	*Challenges and Limitations*	*Future Prospects*
Machine Learning (ML) for Drug Design	ML models analyze large chemical and biological datasets to predict drug properties and optimize lead compounds.	Deep Chem, Chem Prop, QSAR Too lbox, IBM Watson Drug Discovery	Accelerates drug discovery, improves hit identification, reduces costs	Requires high-quality datasets, potential biases in predictions	AI-powered automation for ultra-rapid screening and lead optimization
Deep Learning (DL) in Drug Development	DL algorithms analyze complex biological interactions, structure-activity relationships (SARs), and drug efficacy.	Alpha Fold, Deep Chem, Atom Net, Bio BERT	Enhances target identification, predicts novel drug candidates, improves accuracy	Computationally expensive, requires large datasets, interpretability challenges	Integration with quantum computing for better predictive accuracy
Generative AI for Molecular Design	AI-powered generative models create novel drug-like molecules based on target properties.	Insilico Medicine, GENTRL, Chem GAN, REINVENT, Mol GAN	Accelerates lead discovery, enhances chemical diversity, optimizes drug properties	May generate non-druggable molecules, requires experimental validation	AI-driven iterative design with real-time feedback loops
Natural Language Processing (NLP) in Biomedical Research	NLP extracts insights from biomedical literature, clinical trials, and patents for drug discovery.	Bio BERT, Sci BERT, IBM Watson, PubMed BERT	Automates knowledge extraction, enhances literature mining, improves clinical trial design	Contextual accuracy limitations, requires domain-specific training	AI-powered real-time analysis of biomedical literature for novel insights
Reinforcement Learning (RL) for Drug Optimization	RL models iteratively refine drug candidates by optimizing molecular properties.	Deep Drug, Mol DQN, REINVENT, Alpha Fold-RL	Enhances molecular design, optimizes pharmacokinetics and toxicity profiles	Requires extensive training time, risk of generating unrealistic molecules	AI-driven adaptive drug optimization for precision medicine

Machine Learning (ML) for Drug Design

Drug discovery today heavily relies on ML because this technology accesses large datasets for biological and chemical information to develop significant relationships and understandings [10]. The categories of ML models consist of supervised learning and unsupervised learning and RL which support different research needs within pharmaceutical operations.

Supervised learning finds prevalent application in predictive modeling through training of AI algorithms that work with datasets which contain drug-target interaction information. These models let scientists determine novel compound effectiveness and safety by recognizing biological activity patterns between chemical and structural features. The application of ML resulted in an improved method for analyzing small molecule interactions with protein targets which encouraged scientists to develop better drug prospects [7].

Unsupervised learning focuses on analyzing unstructured dataset collections while the task lacks defined labels. Researchers find this method beneficial to cluster comparable compounds as well as detect new biomarkers while establishing previously undetected disease-drug linkages. The combination analysis of genomic and transcriptomic and proteomic and metabolomic data through AI leads to discovery of hidden patterns which drive progress in personalized medicine [11].

Drugs benefit from dynamic optimization through RL because this method let AI models build better drug structures through experiments which enhance therapeutic characteristics. The continuous development of drug candidates through RL algorithms extends into large chemical domains to achieve highly desirable qualities which include pharmaceutical potency combined with absorption efficiency and reduced toxicology. Through its self-learning skill, AI produces creative drug designs which traditional screening practices would never produce [12].

Deep Learning (DL) in Drug Development

Drug discovery has seen a breakthrough with DL which belongs to the ML family because it allows analyzing complex patterns alongside predicting medicinal properties. The pharmaceutical sector achieves substantial results through DL processing by working with high-dimensional biological data formats, such as molecular structures as well as genetic sequences and medical images [13].

A particular decline in image-based drug screening has occurred because of convolutional neural networks (CNNs). CNNs enable automated cellular response detection through analysis of microscopy images that contain morphological indications of exposure to potential drug compounds. High-content screening assays operate faster due to adopting this technology which allows for better drug candidate identification [14].

Recurrent neural networks (RNNs) possess a dedicated structure that processes data sequences which enables them to run biological time-series data analysis of gene expression patterns and metabolic pathways as well as pharmacokinetic profiles. RNNs acquire knowledge of biological process duration through their temporal capabilities which enables scientists to optimize dosage and forecast toxicity effects in drugs.

The field of drug-protein interaction prediction experiences new developments from transformer models that have captured attention during the recent period. The AI architecture uses self-attention analysis to process intricate molecular relationships with outstanding accuracy [15]. The contextual patterns transformers identify among molecules enhance virtual screening methods, thus creating better conditions for drug discovery.

Generative AI for Molecular Design

Drug discovery became more revolutionary through generative AI technology because it created new pathways for de novo generating drug-like molecules. Drug development under traditional processes needs to examine extensive chemical collections through time-consuming and expensive laboratory screening. Using generative model algorithms enables scientists to build brand new molecular structures which the AI systems optimize through their design algorithms [16].

Generative adversarial networks (GANs) function as one of the top approaches within generative AI frameworks. GANs train dual network systems which produce substance generations then assess their credibility to develop optimized compounds that fulfill specific properties. The discovery of molecules with superior drug-likeness and bioactivity became possible through this method [17].

The applicability of variational autoencoders (VAEs) enables scientists to structure their chemical space exploration effectively during the generative AI process. VAEs transform molecular data into condensed space by learning encoding patterns which permits the generation of new molecular samples for subsequent optimization. Virtual compound generation has benefited from this method because AI automatically improves drug candidates through predefined pharmacological standards.

When AI-driven de novo drug design systems operate pharmaceutical institutions can investigate chemical entities which existing databases do not contain, thus helping develop unique medications for tough and infrequent diseases [18].

Natural Language Processing (NLP) in Biomedical Research

NLP technology stands as a crucial instrument for extracting beneficial clinical insights from extensive biomedical publications as well as electronic healthcare documentation and trial documentation. The use of AI algorithms for text analysis enables scientists to quickly find appropriate research findings, thus keeping them in the loop about modern drug discovery developments.

AI-based literature mining represented by NLP is an essential application because it utilizes automated scanners to identify concealed patterns of drug-disease-pathway relationships within medical literature and patent databases and scientific publications. The automated assessment method decreases literary review time while making research teams more effective at finding drug candidates.

The prediction of adverse drug reactions (ADRs) depends heavily on NLP functionality. Medical texts written without structure, including physician notes and patient reviews, serve as AI input to detect drug safety hazards and potential toxicity phenomena at an early stage [19]. The ability of these systems enables regulatory institutions to execute rapid interventions which protect patients from adverse circumstances.

The drug repurposing methods that utilize NLP-based AI can detect multiple potential therapeutic uses for existing medical products. NLP systems process clinical trial information combined with published research findings and patient results to discover new drug-treatment relationships which speeds up approved medicine applications for different treatment areas [20].

Reinforcement Learning (RL) for Drug Optimization

The field of RL provides industries with an efficient tool to optimize drug product developments and clinical trial methodology designs and device dosing systems. RL functions differently than typical optimization approaches because it obtains information from actual field data which it uses to enhance its decision-making algorithms throughout its operational period.

The combination process of drug formulation components becomes more efficient through AI-guided RL models which override drug bioavailability together with solubility and stability improvements. The predictive capabilities of RL create models to identify the most advantageous formulation combinations between performance improvement and adverse effect reduction [21].

The adaptive clinical trial design transforms through the application of RL. The standard methods used in clinical trials create strict parameters which results in wasted time and productivity problems during drug testing phases. The AI-driven RL system modifies all trial conditions, including patient test standards and medication timing together with therapeutic dosage options by processing immediate test subject responses. The adaptive approach delivers better efficiency to trials with simultaneously reduced research expenses and shortens time needed for new drug approvals [22].

AI-Powered Computational Tools for Drug Discovery

The application of AI throughout drug discovery promotes better efficiency within the pharmaceutical sector at reduced costs with enhanced accuracy. The integration of AI through computational tools builds upon traditional drug research by permitting fast testing of potential medicines and improved understanding of substance interactions and better control of clinical experiment cycles. The tools use ML and DL and other AI-driven approaches to process extensive datasets for detecting valuable compounds which facilitate quick discovery of new medications [23]. The chapter discusses how essential AI computational tools reshape drug discovery with a focus on molecular docking as well as in silico toxicology along with structural biology, HTS, clinical trial optimization, and drug repurposing (Table 2.2).

Table 2.2 AI-Powered Computational Tools for Drug Discovery

Topic	*Description*	*Examples*	*Key Benefits*	*Challenges and Limitations*	*Future Prospects*
Molecular Docking and Virtual Screening Platforms	AI-driven docking predicts drug binding affinity to target proteins, accelerating hit identification.	AutoDock, Glide, SwissDock, GOLD, DockThor, MOE, Schrödinger Suite	Reduces time and cost of hit identification, enhances accuracy	Requires high computational power, may produce false positives	Integration with AI/ML for more precise docking predictions
In Silico Toxicology and Pharmacokinetics Predictions	AI predicts ADMET properties, reducing the need for early stage animal testing.	pkCSM, ADMET Predictor, ProTox-II, SwissADME, Toxtree, Lazar, DeepTox	Improves drug safety assessment, minimizes late stage failures	Accuracy depends on training data quality, limited applicability for novel compounds	More refined deep learning models for personalized toxicity predictions
Bioinformatics and Structural Biology Tools	AI analyzes genomic, proteomic, and structural data to identify potential drug targets.	AlphaFold, Rosetta, SwissSidechain, PDBbind, ModRefiner, FoldX, ChimeraX	Advances understanding of protein structures, accelerates target identification	Structural prediction accuracy may vary, requires large datasets	Integration with quantum computing for enhanced accuracy
AI in High-Throughput Screening (HTS)	AI models analyze large HTS datasets to prioritize promising compounds and reduce false positives.	DeepChem, ChemProp, DeepScreen, ChemNet, MolAICal, QSAR Toolbox	Increases efficiency, reduces cost of large-scale screening	Requires extensive training datasets, potential biases	AI-powered automation for ultra-rapid screening
AI for Clinical Trial Optimization	AI improves trial design, patient recruitment, and biomarker discovery for efficiency.	IBM Watson for Drug Discovery, Trials.ai, Saama AI, Antidote Match, Deep6 AI	Enhances success rates, reduces trial costs and timelines	Ethical concerns, data privacy issues, potential biases	AI-driven adaptive trial designs and real-time monitoring
AI-Driven Drug Repurposing Approaches	AI finds new therapeutic uses for existing drugs using big data and deep learning.	BenevolentAI, DeepDrug, CANDO, GENTrep, DrugBank AI, RepurposeDB	Reduces development time and cost, increases success rates	Data dependency, regulatory challenges	AI-driven network pharmacology for multi-disease drug repurposing

(Continued)

Table 2.2 (Continued)

Topic	*Description*	*Examples*	*Key Benefits*	*Challenges and Limitations*	*Future Prospects*
Generative AI for Drug Design	AI models generate nove drug-like molecules with desired properties	Insilico Medicine, ChemGAN, GENTRL, REINVENT, MolGAN	Accelerates lead compound discovery, enhances molecular diversity	Risk of generating non-druggable molecules, validation challenges	AI-guided de novo drug design with real-time feedback loops
AI-Driven Target Identification and Validation	AI integrates omics data and pathway analysis to identify novel drug targets.	DeepTarget, OpenTargets, Pharos, TargetNet, TIN-X	Enhances target specificity, reduces off-target effects	Requires high-quality datasets, may have false positives	AI-driven precision target identification using multimodal data
AI for Precision Medicine	AI personalizes drug therapies based on patient-specific data.	Tempus, Foundation Medicine, DeepVariant, IBM Watson Genomics	Improves treatment outcomes, minimizes adverse effects	Ethical concerns, data privacy, high implementation costs	AI-powered real-time personalized treatment recommendations
AI-Enabled Biomarker Discovery	AI identifies disease biomarkers using multi-omics and imaging data.	Qlucore Omics Explorer, BioXcel, DeepMind AlphaFold, DeepBiomarker	Enables early disease detection, improves targeted therapy	Requires validation in clinical settings, complex regulatory pathways	AI-driven real-time biomarker monitoring and validation
Quantum Computing in Drug Discovery	Quantum AI simulates molecular interactions at a quantum level.	IBM Quantum, Google Quantum AI, Qubit Pharmaceuticals, D-Wave Leap	Enhances drug design accuracy, enables simulations of complex systems	Expensive technology, requires significant expertise	Scalable quantum AI for large-scale molecular simulations
AI for Formulation Development	AI predicts drug solubility, stability, and optimal delivery methods.	FormulatorAI, Simulations Plus, Cresset Flare, PharmAI	Optimizes drug formulation, improves bioavailability	Limited by available formulation datasets, regulatory challenges	AI-driven predictive formulation for next-generation drug delivery systems

Molecular Docking and Virtual Screening Platforms

Molecular docking and virtual screening represent essential drug discovery methods which predict minimal molecule behaviors toward biological targets especially proteins and enzymes. Computed docking algorithms powered by AI have introduced both fast speed and precise accuracy to these predictions, thus enabling scientists to screen large collections of biological compounds effectively [24].

Traditional physical methods within molecular docking calculations use DL frameworks to boost docking prediction speed while improving accuracy rates for binding affinity predictions. AI models derive their understanding from massive protein-ligand bond databases to successfully spot compounds that present top therapeutic properties. Attractive drug-target binding predictions see enhanced reliability when AI-based molecular simulations include protein movement alongside solvent interactions with dynamic molecular bond activities [25].

Expert researchers have achieved a critical advancement with the combination of AI-quantum hybrid systems used for molecular simulations. Quantum computing systems that team up with AI algorithms enable scientists to develop atomically detailed precise molecular modeling methods. The advanced simulation methods enable more precise examination of complex molecular interactions to produce optimized drug candidates which exhibit stronger binding ability and lower toxicity while improving how the drug gets absorbed in the body. The method shows great potential in developing pharmaceutical options for difficult molecular structures found in disorders, including cancer and neurodegenerative diseases [26].

In Silico Toxicology and Pharmacokinetics Predictions

Drug development needs thorough evaluation of both safety aspects and drug absorption characteristics for prospective drug candidates. AI implements high-accuracy predictive models for in silico toxicology and pharmacokinetics (PK) evaluations of drug absorption, distribution, metabolism, excretion, and toxicity (ADMET) properties.

AI-driven ADMET prediction models examine the chemical composition of molecules to determine their human body response patterns. The integrated system uses preclinical and clinical study data to estimate solubility permeability and metabolic stability and side effects potency. The toxicity risk evaluation done by AI algorithms enables researchers to remove dangerous compounds before significant development stages [1].

AI models that assess drug safety and risks employ DL frameworks to make predictions about adverse effects using chemical information combined with biological data along with drug toxicity records from the past. The implementation of AI-powered toxicological models helps drug safety evaluation by recognizing possible adverse events before clinical trials, thus minimizing the probability of late stage drug failure. The organization of drug candidates becomes more efficient through this approach by both saving resources and selecting superior candidates for clinical trial assessment [27].

Bioinformatics and Structural Biology Tools

Bioinformatics along with structural biology has benefited substantially from AI due to its ability to identify protein 3D shapes and how they bond with pharmaceutical compounds. The discovery of new drugs heavily depends on protein structure prediction since the actual shapes and structural arrangements of proteins define their biological actions as well as their drug response patterns.

The field had a significant advancement because AI technology produced predictive tools for protein structure modeling through AlphaFold and RoseTTAFold. DL models have revolutionized structural biology through their ability to determine protein structures precisely at an atomic resolution. Researches utilize protein structure knowledge to produce medication that locks onto particular disease proteins, thus creating better therapeutic outcomes [28].

DL models are used to process genomic and proteomic data in order to analyze extremely large biological datasets. AI algorithms detect multiple relationships between genes and drugs and disease markers and treatment possibilities through analyzing complex genomic sequences and protein information. The application of this method reinforces precision medicine methods because health providers match medicines to unique patient genetics for better results and decreased adverse side effects.

AI in High-Throughput Screening (HTS)

Drug discovery utilizes HTS as a critical process for conducting rapid biological activity tests on numerous chemical compounds. AI has transformed HTS systems through automated operations and better data evaluation and predictive models [29].

Phenotypic screening performance has increased through AI-driven cell image analytical systems for detecting drug-treatment responses in cells. DL models at an advanced level analyze detailed microscopy images through which they detect faint morphological cell variations of samples tested for new drug candidates. The AI-powered method enhances both screening speed and precision of phenotypic tests leading to faster antivirus compound identification.

High-throughput drug combination screening utilizing AI performs analyses to determine favorable drug interactions. Programmed AI systems examine extensive drug response records to create predictions about drug pairings that yield optimal treatment results mainly for treating cancer and infectious conditions. Things improve when AI optimizes drug pair combinations because it makes treatment more effective while decreasing the chances of wasting medications [30].

AI for Clinical Trial Optimization

The execution of clinical trials constitutes an extremely expensive and lengthy segment in the pharmaceutical development process. The optimization power of AI includes improving three key areas of clinical trials through better patient recruitment along with trial design and patient stratification processes.

AI-based patient stratification together with recruitment models perform analysis on genetic data, medical histories and biomarker profiles to pick eligible participants for clinical studies. The precise participant selection in this method speeds up research activities and leads to superior patient results and fewer participants leaving trials. Predictive models enable AI to determine the appropriate patient selection that speeds up the drug approval process [31].

AI digital twins represent an advanced innovation which operates in clinical trials. Therapeutic digital twins represent digital versions of patients which mimic actual disease developments and medication responses. ACI technology enables scientists to develop individualized simulation models which assist researchers in drug effect evaluations before starting clinical trials on actual patients. The implementation of this method leads to decreased expenses while improving test performance with better protection for patients.

AI-Driven Drug Repurposing Approaches

The adoption of AI technology enables researchers to identify medications from existing therapeutic drugs for alternative disease treatments. The process proves advantageous because it results in both shorter development periods and lower production expenses as opposed to commencing fresh drug development.

GNNs function as drug-drug interaction prediction systems through analysis of intricate medical relationships among drugs and their linked entities, including proteins and diseases. AI models that process wide biomedical datasets assist pharmaceutical research by identifying possible new therapeutic uses for drugs that currently exist. The molecular-level drug interaction predictions of GNNs succeed in revealing new treatment solutions that science did not detect before [32].

The implementation of DL-based knowledge graphs through AI technology develops complex biological correlations between multiple diseases for drug indication expansion. AI systems optimized through knowledge graphs unite three types of information which includes clinical evidence with genomic and molecular sequencing data to find relationships between medications and disease networks. The use of AI in drug repurposing tasks allows researchers to identify new treatment possibilities which enable them to find medicines for rare illnesses and disorders and emerging diseases [33].

Integration of AI with Emerging Technologies

Speedy advancements in AI technology currently drive drug discovery by executing advanced processes with increased speed while cutting down expenses and generating more accurate predictions. AI operates at limited effectiveness when encountering the extensive molecular patterns and evolving data security challenges as well as genetic processes. New solutions emerge from the combination of AI systems with quantum computing and blockchain together with federated learning and CRISPR-based gene editing technology approaches to solve these problems. The combination of multiple fields of study produces better computational power alongside data protection mechanisms and optimized genetic transformation which speeds up precise drug development [34].

AI and Quantum Computing in Drug Discovery

The advancement of AI technology enables drug discovery through three essential elements which include predictive analytics and molecular modeling and biomarker identification. The complexity present in molecular interactions as well as chemical phenomena at the quantum level makes it challenging for traditional computing systems to handle these processes effectively. Quantum computing solves the limitations by performing complex parallel processing operations. The connection between quantum computing systems with AI technology brings fresh discoveries to molecular simulations together with drug screening techniques and chemical structure optimization [22].

Quantum-AI Hybrid Models for Molecular Simulations

Understandings of protein-ligand associations together with enzyme procedures depend on molecular simulations as well as drug-target binding strength calculations. The molecular modeling techniques MD and DFT operate with extensive computational needs while using approximate solutions. The combination of quantum computing with AI delivers improved atomic level quantum mechanical interaction modeling for these simulations. Programs based on AI together with quantum operations predict the natural behaviors of molecules while finding better ways to execute chemical processes and measure substance interactions with their intended biological targets. Drugs become more effective when designed with this dual method since it gives accurate predictions about molecular action which gives rise to targeted treatments [35].

Quantum Machine Learning for Faster Drug Screening

Drug discovery necessitates the evaluation of large chemical information libraries in order to detect potential drug candidates. The speedup of AI-based virtual screening tests depends on traditional computing platforms unable to handle complex quantum mechanical features. QML improves intelligence capabilities through quantum patterns detection and feature process while analyzing extensive datasets with its algorithm power. The new drug screening models shortens computational duration; thus, researchers can assess millions of compounds with better efficiency. Quantum AI-based drug screening identifies new potential therapeutic compounds among small molecules as well as peptides and biologics through its ability to decrease false discovery results during drug discovery evaluation [36].

Blockchain and Federated Learning in AI-Driven Drug Discovery

The implementation of AI drug discovery depends on patient data and genomic information and clinical trial datasets while creating security and privacy risks together with ethical concerns. The combination of blockchain technology with federated learning implements protection solutions for pharmaceutical research through their establishment of secure decentralized AI models which protect privacy [37].

Quantum-AI Hybrid Models for Molecular Simulations

The analysis of protein-ligand binding interactions and enzyme processes and medications toward their targets requires molecular simulations as a basic scientific tool. Molecular modeling techniques using both molecular dynamics and density functional theory require powerful computing systems as well as work with variable approximations. These simulations benefit from quantum computing combined with AI because they achieve exact quantum mechanical atomic level interaction modeling. Quantum algorithms powered by AI technology enables scientists to map molecular energy pathways as well as enhance chemical transformation and model how drugs interact with biological targets. The combination of these approaches streamlines drug development because it produces accurate predictions of molecular activities that guide improved therapeutic interventions [38].

Quantum Machine Learning for Faster Drug Screening

Drug discovery necessitates the evaluation of large chemical information libraries in order to detect potential drug candidates. The speedup process in drug discovery through virtual screening relies on AI technology yet standard computing faces limitations when handling sophisticated quantum mechanical properties. QML improves intelligence capabilities through quantum patterns detection and feature process while analyzing extensive datasets with its algorithm power [39]. The new drug screening models shortens computational duration; thus, researchers can assess millions of compounds with better efficiency. Through quantum AI-based drug screening, laboratories can detect pharmaceutical agents with a therapeutic value which reduces their pipeline testing errors (Figure 2.2).

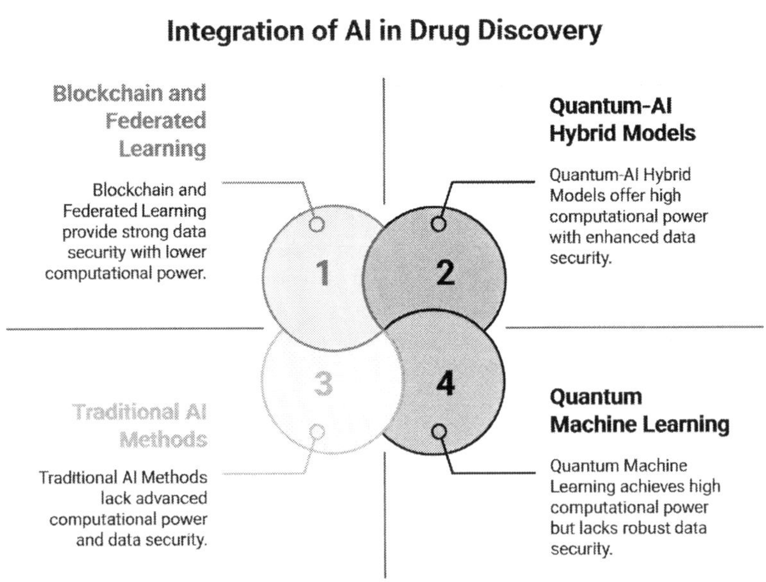

Figure 2.2 Integration of AI in Drug Discovery

Blockchain and Federated Learning in AI-Driven Drug Discovery

AI-driven drug discovery depends increasingly on patient information and genomic results and clinical trial findings yet leads to security and privacy and ethical challenges in data management. Both blockchain and federated learning systems deliver protected and privacy-protected AI model solutions which address drug discovery security requirements in pharmaceutical research [14].

AI-Guided CRISPR Gene Editing for Precision Medicine

Scientists can use CRISPR technology to edit genes specifically but require a comprehensive method for selecting appropriate target sites in the genome. The prediction of highly effective and protected CRISPR target sites emerges from the analysis of extensive genomic data performed by AI-based DL models. Genetic variations together with mutation patterns and biological pathways exist in these models to guarantee that CRISPR modifications create the anticipated therapeutic effects without unwanted side effects. The combination of CRISPR technology with AI allows scientists to develop specific genetic treatments for healthy patients suffering from diseases, such as sickle cell anemia, cystic fibrosis along with hereditary cancers through precise medicine approaches [13].

AI in Genome-Wide Off-Target Prediction

The use of CRISPR-based gene editing exposes patients to major risks because unintended genetic changes emerge at points different from the target region potentially causing dangerous consequences. AI predictive systems incorporate bioinformatics and DL methods to analyze guide RNA (gRNA) performance and detect gRNA-targeted interactions which could lead to harmful consequences. AI methods that examine entire genomes enhance CRISPR precision which lowers the possibility of disturbed genetic sequences. The combination of AI technologies enables experts to develop ideal CRISPR constructs which perform gene modifications precisely and protect the system from unwanted side effects. Modernized approaches play a central role to guarantee the clinical safety together with therapeutic effectiveness of CRISPR-based therapeutic methods [40].

Challenges and Ethical Considerations in AI-Driven Drug Discovery

The pharmaceutical industry uses AI for drug development innovation alongside financial and prediction improvement. The implementation of AI technologies brings forward different obstacles and moral concerns that need resolution to create responsible systems. Healthcare professionals face various difficulties when implementing AI systems because these tools present risks to personal information privacy and security along with AI model biases while also creating regulatory compliance challenges together with moral issues related to AI decision-making in clinical testing and customized medicine. Such critical matters need resolution to make the most of AI while protecting both patient rights and study integrity and public trust in AI-based healthcare developments [41].

Data Privacy, Security, and Bias in AI Models

Drug discovery using AI depends mainly on enormous biomedical datasets consisting of genomic data together with EHRs and molecular structures as well as clinical trial information. Data privacy together with security concerns emerge as major issues due to the use of these datasets in AI predictive functions. Medical and genomic records along with other patient data possess high sensitivity levels so unauthorized breaches and unauthorized access result in identity theft or financial fraud or medical information misuse. AI depends on patient data learning to continuously develop so the risk increases for unintentional exposure of personally identifiable information (PII), thus requiring robust data protection protocols [1].

The main obstacle during drug discovery powered by AI arises when AI models absorb biases contained in previous datasets. Computational predictions made by AI systems tend to become either deceptive or detrimental toward minority user groups when training material does not represent diverse populations. Drug efficiency prediction models operate best for a specific population type but they tend to provide limited accuracy across various population subgroups so drug distribution and efficacy levels become inconsistent between groups. Researches need to provide AI models with diverse representative datasets but also need to use bias detection algorithms together with fairness-aware ML techniques. The disclosure of AI decision processes remains vital since it lets researchers and regulators detect biases which must be fixed prior to AI-drug candidates advancing toward clinical trials [4].

The scarcity of available data constitutes a critical issue during AI model training especially when researchers need to work with rare diseases and new drug objectives with insufficient patient information. The precision of AI predictions depends on extensive high-quality datasets, yet numerous diseases particularly rare diseases cannot access adequate data needed for correct forecasting. Unreliable predictions along with restricted AI effectiveness for drug discovery emerge when there is not enough data available. The scarcity of available data requires scientists to use computational methods that include GANs or VAEs for synthetic data generation as well as transfer learning between related diseases and federated learning methods which combine distributed institutions to train AI models securely without losing privacy capabilities. The approaches develop AI models that gain higher applicability across different situations and lead to more effective drug research while avoiding the violation of patient data confidentiality [42].

Regulatory and Compliance Challenges

Drug discovery programs enabled by AI technology need to respect the exacting requirements defined by world health authorities, including the U.S. Food and Drug Administration (FDA), European Medicines Agency (EMA), and International Council for Harmonisation of Technical Requirements for Pharmaceuticals for Human Use (ICH). The current regulatory procedures aimed at standard drugs were made primarily for traditional drug creation systems but fail to match AI research speed. AI drug discovery receives regulatory hurdles from the absence of standardized validation protocols which creates unknowns in approval examinations that prevent pharmaceutical companies from obtaining clearance for their produced candidates [43].

AI-generated molecules face major regulatory hurdles because proper guidelines do not exist for these new molecules. AI-generated compounds containing new original chemical compounds require regulatory agencies to design fresh assessment protocols to determine both safety performance and risk characteristics of such compounds. AI-based models function as impenetrable systems which create difficulties for regulators to determine the drug candidate selection process. The development of XAI methods by researchers focuses on enhancing regulatory compliance since these techniques enable AI systems to generate understandable explanations for their predicted outcomes [44].

Good Machine Learning Practices (GMLP) compliance represents a vital element for launching AI-based drug development approaches. GMLP provides uniform guidelines for building AI models as well as testing and implementing them in healthcare applications. Drugs detected through AI-assisted searches become more transparent and can be reproduced more easily along with gaining regulatory trust which speeds up approval processes. Overcoming regulatory barriers during AI drug discovery requires organizations to establish early contact with regulatory agencies while documenting model development comprehensively and forming teams of clinicians and specialists and experts in regulation [45].

Ethical AI in Personalized Medicine and Clinical Trials

The benefits of AI to personalized medicine emerge through using individual-genetic and metabolic and life-style factors to create targeted drug treatments for patients. AI-based personalized medicine generates ethical boundaries about how patients control their health decisions and consent to treatment methods and computerized medical choices. A vital moral problem involves confirming patients fully grasp how AI builds treatment suggestions as well as the potential dangers along with uncertainties related to such decisions. AI models may elect to suggest treatment alternatives using complex data algorithms which healthcare providers and patients cannot easily understand and simplify, thus creating problems of placing excessive reliance on decisions derived from AI systems. The solution requires elevated explainability with transparent AI management of medical diagnoses and treatment recommendations so both patients and healthcare providers get sufficient information for making decisions [46].

AI technology currently helps clinical trials by managing patient selection processes and helps optimize clinical trial protocols and tracks therapeutic results throughout the study. The increased efficiency which results from AI implementation causes both ethical concerns about data fairness along with integrity issues. The selection criteria for participants in clinical trials that use AI systems need to maintain free from biases which prevent particular groups from participating. The AI-controlled monitoring system needs to maintain stringent data integrity standards to stop intentional result alteration. Medical authorities have to develop comprehensive guidelines that determine proper use of AI within clinical trials which must prioritize both accuracy and patient security [27].

The practice of using AI for drug discovery requires detailed evaluation of two vital ethical elements: liability as well as accountability. Medical organizations face difficulties in establishing accountable parties regarding drug candidate safety failures that emerge from AI systems. The AI developers and the pharmaceutical company and regulatory agencies and medication providers all lack clear accountability relations. AI accountability frameworks need to be formulated under law for drug development and medical choices to enable proper use of ethical AI systems in healthcare [20].

Future Directions in AI-Powered Drug Discovery

The pharmaceutical field experiences substantial change because of AI drug discovery speedup methods that develop advanced drug development methods alongside precise solutions and cost-saving approaches. The evolution of advanced AI systems currently leads to numerous emerging advances which will substantially revolutionize drug discovery processes. The future directions of AI-powered drug discovery will witness three aspects: multi-omics analysis development, self-teaching AI systems acceptance and distributed AI networks establishment and next-level AI-powered drug development at an individual level. These technological advancements establish routes to better and more effective drug discovery operations promoting improved healthcare results for global patients [47].

Advancements in AI-Powered Multi-Omics Analysis

Athens-based Clinical Research Center serves as central medical research facility to lead precision medicine through analyzing genomic and transcriptomic and proteomic and metabolomic and epigenomic data. The extensive use of AI makes it possible for scientists to find meaningful insights in complex datasets which leads to new drug targets while allowing them to predict disease path and develop personalized medications. ML with DL models operates on vast multi-omics datasets to discover both biomarkers linked to particular diseases as well as provide data-centric drug discovery bases [48].

AI-powered multi-omics analysis has reached a new milestone by merging various data types, including patient genetic data and protein relationships with metabolic systems together. AI models reveal undiscovered relationships that link genetic variations to disease phenotypes which speed up the process of finding drug targets and identifying new drug candidates. Through predictive modeling AI systems monitor genetic mutation effects on drugs, thus helping pharmaceutical development of precise medicines that reduce side effects. AI progress will enable better understanding of combined omics datasets while propelling advances in precise medical care and expediting the development of fresh medicine candidates [49].

The Rise of Self-Learning AI Models for Drug Development

AI algorithms used through traditional drug discovery methods depend on previously collected datasets together with human-manually applied labels to predict outcomes. AI systems used for drug discovery will reach their peak potential with the development of self-teaching AI platforms that build knowledge bases autonomously through real-world data analysis. Modern RL and unsupervised learning systems develop through time while generating better predictions along with fresh knowledge from these processes.

AI systems trained in self-learning will process experimental outcomes along with clinical trial findings and actual patient responses to update drug candidate estimates automatically. Self-learning algorithms through RL optimize pharmaceutical product specifications by conducting multiple model simulations then learning from observed system responses. The adaptive AI models enable discovery of new chemical structures that hold therapeutic potential which extends the drug discovery strategies above traditional methods [22].

AI systems that learn by themselves help decrease drug development failures because they detect potential setbacks during earlier stages of development. AI models that receive and update their knowledge base through experimental findings achieve higher decision accuracy which lowers expenses from late stage clinical trial failures. Advanced self-learning AI systems will establish a critical function in optimizing pharmaceutical discovery together with pharmaceutical development procedures.

Decentralized AI Platforms for Global Drug Discovery Collaborations

The field of AI drug discovery continues a shift toward decentralized teamwork models which bring pharmaceutical companies academic institutions and investigators to join global drug development collaborations. Decentralized AI systems that use federated learning together with blockchain dual managing technology enable many institutions to analyze data collectively while preventing raw medical information exposure. This system ensures both safety and confidentiality of patient data [12].

AI models benefit from federated learning because the system permits training of models with distributed data across separate institutions which maintains all sensitive information within its originating location. This method enables extensive research cooperations through AI with patient data security retained. Researcher access to decentralized AI networks increases their ability to obtain extensive patient data which produces better AI prediction results across diverse patients.

The data protection features of blockchain technology support superior decentralized AI partnerships through permanent records and unambiguous details and trackable information. Smart contracts on blockchain establish secure transactions for AI-driven drug discovery which also supports ethical data-sharing practices for verification purposes. AIT platforms with distributed networks demonstrate capability to speed up drug research through combined worldwide expert capabilities and data management systems that protect regulatory rules and protect information security protocols (Figure 2.3).

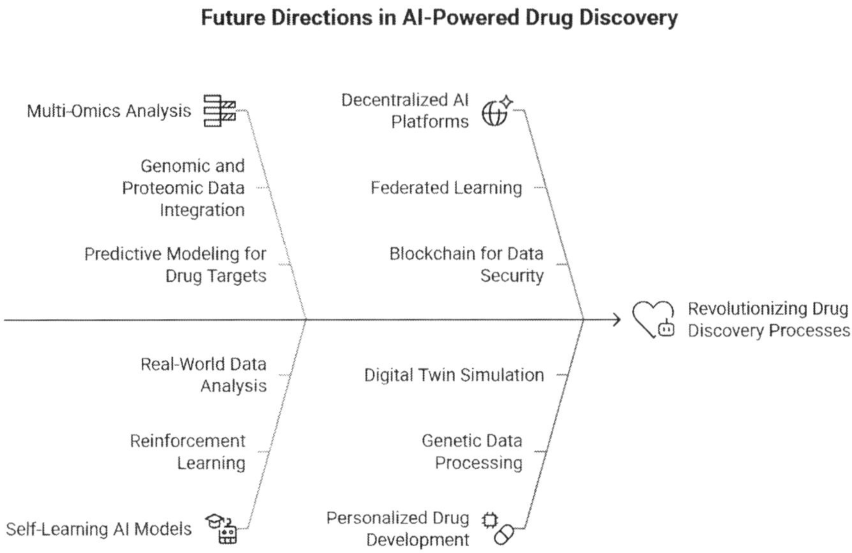

Figure 2.3 Future Directions in AI-Powered Drug Discovery

Next-Generation AI-Powered Personalized Drug Development

The advancement of precision medicine will benefit from AI which develops customized therapeutic solutions that address patients individually. AI systems process genetic data alongside metabolic route information and life patterns to create specific drug therapies that deliver superior results and reduce negative side effects. A personalized treatment method shows maximum benefit for difficult health conditions, including cancer along with neurodegenerative disorders and rare inherited diseases, because standard treatment plans generally prove ineffective for these conditions.

The application of DL models in drug development leads to predictions of specific drug responses for individual patients. AI represents a model for examining drug-protein interactions that assists health systems to choose optimum medical treatments for individual patients. The optimization of drug formulations receives help from AI systems when they process drug absorption and distribution together with metabolism and excretion (ADME) characteristics across various genetic backgrounds [50].

Medical experts use AI technology to create digital twins representing individual patients which enables simulation of therapeutic responses before starting treatments. The creation of digital twins enables scientists to evaluate numerous therapeutic plans through simulated virtual models which minimize the conventional testing process in precision medicine treatment. Next-generation drug development using AI processing of individual patient data will transform healthcare delivery by providing unique biological treatments that precisely match healthcare needs.

Conclusion

The Transformative Role of AI in Drug Discovery

The drug discovery field now depends heavily on AI as an innovative tool that makes traditional procedures better and speeds up the therapeutic development process. Medical pipelines dedicated to drug research benefit greatly from AI-oriented approaches like DL and ML and NLP technology which enhances both their operational accuracy and success rates while facilitating improved efficiency. AI demonstrates vital capabilities in molecular docking systems while performing drug-target virtual screening evaluations and predicting drug-target association outcomes. The use of AI for bioinformatics combined with structural biology tools helps scientists analyze complex biological data which supports the discovery of new drug candidates [51].

AI through its automation of screening procedures shortens drug discovery durations and lowers overall expenses. Through dedicated AI algorithms researchers get help in processing huge multi-omics datasets which reveal new biomarkers and help segment patients into groups. Modern pharmaceutical sciences benefit strongly from the use of AI which enables drug interaction modeling while predicting adverse reactions together with better clinical trial design optimization. AI advancement expects to expand innovation in drug discovery through its integration with quantum computing along with blockchain technology and CRISPR gene editing systems.

Future Implications and AI's Potential in Revolutionizing Pharmaceuticals

The pharmaceutical sector faces an exciting future because advancements will continue toward self-learning AI systems together with decentralized AI platforms and multi-omics data consolidation. Medical drug development using AI approaches will increase precision and allow for patient-specific solutions that deliver effective treatments with reduced side effects.

The main benefit of AI in pharmaceuticals consists of its ability to create personalized medicinal approaches. Healthcare professionals now implement AI models that handle patient-specific genetic and clinical data to generate made-to-measure treatment strategies. It is predicted that this advancement could transform disease treatments specifically in cancer patients because personal medicine strategies result in better therapeutic outcomes. AI allows for drug repurposing through existing drug identification for new therapeutic use with the aim of speeding up and lowering the costs for drug approval [41].

The use of AI in predictive toxicology as well as PK modeling and disease progression analysis will lead to better safety and effectiveness in drug development. Through the integration of AI with patient virtual replicas called digital twins healthcare professionals can perform instant drug response simulations to enhance clinical trial development and regulatory approval processes. The combination of blockchain technologies with federated learning models helps AI systems enable secure data exchange across global pharmaceutical companies during drug research efforts.

Software developments in AI will produce fresh drug categories and enact improvements in vaccine work while providing better medical tests. AI implementation needs to follow ethical and regulatory and compliance standards for achieving responsible pharmaceutical research utilization.

The Need for Human-AI Collaboration in Drug Development

Drug discovery advancements through AI technology need human experts to analyze AI output and handle the most important choices. Drug development through AI needs equally powerful collaboration between both human intellect and learning algorithms to succeed. AI can rapidly analyze vast datasets and generate predictions, but human researchers must validate these findings, ensuring their reliability and clinical applicability.

Human-AI partnership plays an essential role to solve ethical issues that include algorithmic bias together with data privacy and regulatory compliance problems. AI models perform with the same accuracy as their foundation datasets do because biases in training data cause frequent inaccurate predictions. AI drug development requires human supervision for ethical compliance and fairness protocols and potential risk management operations.

AI must be implemented by a shared effort between both pharmaceutical scientists and clinicians to work hand in hand with developers and regulatory authorities to ensure a proper integration. The conduct of the FDA, EMA, and ICH must develop collective guidance together with AI expert teams to determine safe and effective application of AI systems in pharmaceutical research [52].

The ongoing evolution of AI technology requires developers to use it for human intelligence enhancement instead of performing human substitution. AI acts as an empowering resource to strengthen human choices in addition to speeding up research along with creating new innovation. Advanced drug discovery will result from AI-analogous cooperation with human experts to generate superior medical treatments and enhanced therapeutic outcomes while enabling precise medical strategies.

References

1. Chen, H., Engkvist, O., Wang, Y., Olivecrona, M., & Blaschke, T. (2018). The rise of deep learning in drug discovery. *Drug Discovery Today*, *23*(6), 1241–1250.
2. Jumper, J., Evans, R., Pritzel, A., Green, T., Figurnov, M., Ronneberger, O., & Hassabis, D. (2021). Highly accurate protein structure prediction with AlphaFold. *Nature*, *596*(7873), 583–589.
3. Schneider, P., Walters, W. P., Plowright, A. T., Sieroka, N., Listgarten, J., Goodnow, R. A., & Segler, M. H. S. (2020). Rethinking drug design in the artificial intelligence era. *Nature Reviews Drug Discovery*, *19*(5), 353–364.
4. Zhavoronkov, A. (2018). Artificial intelligence for drug discovery, biomarker development, and generation of novel chemistry. *Molecular Pharmaceutics*, *15*(10), 4311–4313.
5. Aminabee, S. K., Prabhakar, M. C., Prasad, R. G. S. V., & Lakshmana Rao, A. (2011). Screening the pharmacological activity of cerium oxide nanoparticles in-vitro. *Biomedical and Pharmacology Journal*, *4*(2), 287–289.

6. Zeng, X., Song, X., Ma, T., Pan, X., Zhou, Y., Zhu, H., & Cao, R. (2022). Deep learning predicts drug pharmacokinetics and drug-drug interactions. *Nature Machine Intelligence*, *4*(1), 40–53.
7. Vamathevan, J., Clark, D., Czodrowski, P., Dunham, I., Ferran, E., Lee, G., & Madabhushi, A. (2019). Applications of machine learning in drug discovery and development. *Nature Reviews Drug Discovery*, *18*(6), 463–477.
8. Walters, W. P., & Murcko, M. A. (2020). Artificial intelligence in drug discovery and development. *Future Medicinal Chemistry*, *12*(18), 1647–1652.
9. Yang, X., Wang, Y., Byrne, R., Schneider, G., & Yang, S. (2019). Concepts of artificial intelligence for computer-assisted drug discovery. *Chemical Reviews*, *119*(18), 10520–10594.
10. Aminabee, S. K., Lakshmana Rao, A., Sowmya, K., Nymisha, D., Kusuma Naga Lakshmi, K., Manikanta, K. V. N. S., & Praveen Kumar, P. (2019). Evaluation of analgesic activity of *Ficus palmata*. *Iranian Journal of Pharmaceutical Sciences*, *15*(3), 47–60.
11. Ekins, S., Puhl, A. C., Zorn, K. M., Lane, T. R., Russo, D. P., Klein, J. J., & Freundlich, J. S. (2019). Exploiting machine learning for end-to-end drug discovery and development. *Nature Materials*, *18*(5), 435–441.
12. Merk, D., Friedrich, L., Grisoni, F., & Schneider, G. (2018). De novo design of bioactive small molecules by artificial intelligence. *Molecular Informatics*, *37*(1–2), 1700153.
13. Stokes, J. M., Yang, K., Swanson, K., Jin, W., Cubillos-Ruiz, A., Donghia, N. M., & Collins, J. J. (2020). A deep learning approach to antibiotic discovery. *Cell*, *180*(4), 688–702.e13.
14. Zhavoronkov, A., Ivanenkov, Y. A., Aliper, A., Veselov, M. S., Aladinskiy, V. A., Aladinskaya, A. V., & Zholus, A. (2019). Deep learning enables rapid identification of potent DDR1 kinase inhibitors. *Nature Biotechnology*, *37*(9), 1038–1040.
15. Sadybekov, A. A., Sadybekov, A. V., Liu, Y., Iliopoulos-Tsoutsouvas, C., Huang, X. P., Pickett, J., & Shoichet, B. K. (2022). Synthon-based ligand discovery in virtual libraries of over 11 billion compounds. *Nature*, *601*(7893), 452–459.
16. Aminabee, S. K., Lakshmana Rao, A., & Chinna Eswaraiah, M. (2020). In-vivo antioxidant activity of different fractions of *Indigofera barberi* against paracetamol-induced toxicity in rats. *Turkish Journal of Pharmaceutical Sciences*, *17*(2), 136–140.
17. Grechishnikova, D. (2021). Transformer neural network for protein-specific de novo drug generation as a machine translation problem. *Scientific Reports*, *11*, 321.
18. Tanoli, Z., Alam, Z., Vähä-Koskela, M., Ravikumar, B., Malyutina, A., Jaiswal, A., & Tang, J. (2021). Interactive visual analysis of drugeractive visual analysis of protein-specific de novo drug generation as a machine translation problemdrug repurposing. *Briefings in Bioinformatics*, *22*(2), 189–202.
19. Rifaioglu, A. S., Atas, H., Martin, M. J., Cetin-Atalay, R., Atalay, V., & Dogan, T. (2018). Recent applications of deep learning and machine intelligence on in silico drug discovery: Methods, tools and databases. *Briefings in Bioinformatics*, *20*(5), 1878–1912.
20. Kadurin, A., Nikolenko, S., Khrabrov, K., Aliper, A., & Zhavoronkov, A. (2017). druGAN: An advanced generative adversarial autoencoder model for de novo generation of new molecules with desired molecular properties in silico. *Molecular Pharmaceutics*, *14*(9), 3098–3104.
21. Prasanth, D. S. N. B. K., Aminabee, S. K., Lakshmana Rao, A., Teja, N., Bhargavi, K., Monika, C., Pujitha, B., Sandhya, T., Lalitha, A., & Siva Prasad, P. (2020). Anthelmintic activity of *Mansoa alliacea* against *Pheretima posthuma*: In-vitro and in-silico approach. *Thai Journal of Pharmaceutical Sciences*, *4*(3), 186–196.
22. Elton, D. C., Boukouvalas, Z., Fuge, M. D., & Chung, P. W. (2019). Deep learning for molecular design - A review of the state of the art. *Molecular Systems Design & Engineering*, *4*(4), 828–849.

23. Winter, R., Montanari, F., Noé, F., & Clevert, D. A. (2019). Learning continuous and data-driven molecular descriptors by translating equivalent chemical representations. *Chemical Science*, *10*(6), 1692–1701.
24. Yang, G., Yang, X., Tang, X., & Wu, H. (2022). A review on machine learning for drug discovery: Algorithms, databases, and applications. *Artificial Intelligence Review*, *55*, 3253–3307.
25. Vamathevan, J., Clark, D., Czodrowski, P., Dunham, I., Ferran, E., Lee, G., & Bender, A. (2019). Applications of machine learning in drug discovery and development. *Nature Reviews Drug Discovery*, *18*, 463–477.
26. Prasanth, D. S. N. B. K., Aminabee, S. K., Lakshmana Rao, A., Guntupalli, C., Reddy, A. R., Kulandaivelu, U., Rao, S. N. K., & Rajeshwari, P. (2021). Inhibitory effects of *Mansoa alliacea* in Freundiaceacts of scoverying in drug discovery and developmentases, and applicasilico strategy. *Thai Journal of Pharmaceutical Sciences*, *45*(6), 532–544.
27. Walters, W. P., & Murcko, M. A. (2020). Assessing the impact of generative AI on medicinal chemistry. *Nature Biotechnology*, *38*(2), 143–145.
28. Ching, T., Himmelstein, D. S., Beaulieu-Jones, B. K., Kalinin, A. A., Do, B. T., Way, G. P., & Greene, C. S. (2018). Opportunities and obstacles for deep learning in biology and medicine. *Journal of the Royal Society Interface*, *15*(141), 20170387.
29. Ragoza, M., Hochuli, J., Idrobo, E., Sunseri, J., & Koes, D. R. (2017). Protein–Ligand Scoring with Convolutional Neural Networks Royal Society Interfaceearning in biology. *Journal of Chemical Information and Modeling*, *57*(4), 942–957.
30. Aminabee, S. K., Santhi Krupa, D., Hanumanth Rao, K., Sirisha, V., Anitha Kumari, V., Nagasen, D., Sujiya, B., & Leelavati, T. S. (2023). Pharmacoeconomic analysis of biologic vs. biosimilar therapies in rheumatoid arthritis. *International Journal of Chemical and Biochemical Sciences*, *24*(4), 395–400.
31. Pereira, J. C., Caffarena, E. R., & Dos Santos, C. N. (2016). Boosting docking-based virtual screening with deep learning. *Journal of Chemical Information and Modeling*, *56*(12), 2495–2506.
32. Zhang, Q., Ma, X., Wang, J., & Chen, B. (2021). Applications of artificial intelligence in drug development using real-world data. *Drug Discovery Today*, *26*(6), 1452–1460.
33. Zhou, Z., Kearnes, S., Li, L., Zare, R. N., & Riley, P. (2019). Optimization of molecules via deep reinforcement learning. *Scientific Reports*, *9*, 10752.
34. Wang, Y., Yao, Q., Kwok, J. T., & Ni, L. M. (2020). Generalizing from a few examples: A survey on few-shot learning. *ACM Computing Surveys (CSUR)*, *53*(3), 1–34.
35. Gao, K., Nguyen, D. D., Tu, M., & Wei, G. W. (2021). Generative network complex for drug discovery. *Journal of Computational Chemistry*, *42*(12), 928–943.
36. Leelavati, T. S., Madhavi, S., Kamal, G., Raju, P. V. M., Susmitha, K., Vinod, M., & Aminabee, S. K. (2023). Revolutionizing healthcare delivery: Telemedicinein influence on access and patient satisfaction. *International Journal of Chemical and Biochemical Sciences*, *24*(5), 106–115.
37. Jin, W., Barzilay, R., & Jaakkola, T. (2018). Junction tree variational autoencoder for molecular graph generation. *Proceedings of the 35th International Conference on Machine Learning*, 2323–2332.
38. Huang, K., Fu, T., Gao, W., Zhao, Y., Roohani, Y., Leskovec, J., & Coley, C. W. (2022). Artificial intelligence foundation for therapeutic science. *Nature Chemical Biology*, *18*(10), 1033–1036.
39. Mamoshina, P., Vieira, A., Putin, E., & Zhavoronkov, A. (2016). Applications of deep learning in biomedicine. *Molecular Pharmaceutics*, *13*(5), 1445–1454.
40. Aminabee, S. K., Devi Mallika, K., & Lakshmana Rao, A. (2023). Natural resources in management and treatment of diseases: A review. *Pharma Times*, *55*(11), 7–10.
41. Gómez-Bombarelli, R., Wei, J. N., Duvenaud, D., Hernandez-Lobato, J. M., Sánchez-Lengeling, B., Sheberla, D., & Aspuru-Guzik, A. (2018). Automatic chemical design

using a data-driven continuous representation of molecules. *ACS Central Science*, *4*(2), 268–276.
42. Bender, A., & Cortes-Ciriano, I. (2021). Artificial intelligence in drug discovery: What is realistic, what are illusions? Part 1: Ways to make an impact, and why we are not there yet. *Drug Discovery Today*, *26*(2), 511–524.
43. Ekins, S., Puhl, A. C., Zorn, K. M., Lane, T. R., Russo, D. P., Klein, J. J., & Clark, A. M. (2019). Exploiting machine learning for end-to-end drug discovery and development. *Nature Materials*, *18*(5), 435–441.
44. Aminabee, S. K., & Lakshmana Rao, A. (2024). Computational identification of selected bioactive compounds from *Cedrus deodara* as inhibitors against SARS-CoV-2 main protease: A pharmacoinformatics study. *Indian Drugs*, *61*(2), 78–91.
45. van Westen, G. J., Wegner, J. K., Ijzerman, A. P., & van Vlijmen, H. W. (2011). Proteochemometric modeling as a tool to design selective compounds and for extrapolating to novel targets. *Medicinal Research Reviews*, *31*(3), 447–466.
46. Korotcov, A., Tkachenko, V., Russo, D. P., & Ekins, S. (2017). Comparison of deep learning with multiple machine learning methods and metrics using diverse drug discovery data sets. *Molecular Pharmaceutics*, *14*(12), 4462–4475.
47. Ravi Shankar, K., Aminabee, S. K., Ramana, G., Chenchu Lakshmi, K. N. V., & Indusree, G. (2024). Formulation and evaluation of propranolol hydrochloride floating tablets by 32 factorial design. *International Journal of Drug Delivery Technology*, *14*(4), 2060–2067.
48. Segler, M. H., Kogej, T., Tyrchan, C., & Waller, M. P. (2018). Generating focused molecule libraries for drug discovery with recurrent neural networks. *ACS Central Science*, *4*(1), 120–131.
49. Schneider, G. (2018). Automating drug discovery. *Nature Reviews Drug Discovery*, *17*(2), 97–113.
50. Popova, M., Isayev, O., & Tropsha, A. (2018). Deep reinforcement learning for de novo drug design. *Science Advances*, *4*(7), eaap7885.
51. Blaschke, T., Olivecrona, M., Engkvist, O., Bajorath, J., & Chen, H. (2018). Application of generative autoencoder in de novo molecular design. *Molecular Informatics*, *37*(1–2), 1700123.
52. Brown, N., Fiscato, M., Segler, M. H. S., & Vaucher, A. C. (2019). GuacaMol: Benchmarking models for de novo molecular design. *Journal of Chemical Information and Modeling*, *59*(3), 1096–1108.

3 Data Collection and Management for AI in Drug Discovery

Introduction to Data-Driven AI in Drug Discovery

The advent of Artificial Intelligence (AI) has transformed the landscape of drug discovery, making it more efficient and data-driven. Traditional drug discovery is a complex and resource-intensive process, often requiring years of research and billions of dollars to bring a single drug to market. The success rate of conventional drug development is also low, with many potential candidates failing during preclinical and clinical trials. AI proves to be a forceful instrument for handling these roadblocks by performing substance-target interaction predictions with enormous data quantities to improve drug compounds and help accelerate medical investigations. Powerful machine learning (ML) and deep learning (DL) algorithms operated through massive datasets let researchers discover better drug candidates more swiftly than conventional methods. AI models prove essential for such tasks as they enable accurate property prediction together with disease mechanism modeling while facilitating existing drug transformation to new therapeutic uses [1].

One of the fundamental aspects of AI-driven drug discovery is data availability and management. AI models require extensive datasets to train and learn from, allowing them to recognize patterns, make predictions, and improve decision-making in drug development. The data used in these models can be broadly categorized into structured and unstructured data. The category of structured data includes well-formatted machine-processable information which involves chemical compound databases together with protein structures and high-throughput screening (HTS) results and clinical trial outcomes as well as genomic data. AI algorithms are able to process these systematically arranged datasets without any difficulty. Unstructured data, however, includes scientific literature, research articles, patents, electronic health records (EHRs), and physician notes, which require natural language processing (NLP) techniques to extract meaningful insights. The integration of both structured and unstructured data enhances AI's predictive capabilities and facilitates comprehensive drug discovery models [2].

Despite the potential of AI in drug discovery, the quality of data remains a critical factor in ensuring accurate and meaningful outcomes. High-quality, unbiased datasets are essential for training AI models to produce reliable predictions.

DOI: 10.4324/9781003616177-3

Inadequate data collection methods along with inconsistent information entry and unrecorded or compromised data points results in misdirected drug development predictions which significantly contributes to development failures later in the process. The improvement of data quality uses multiple methods, including strict database management along with preprocessing and validation procedures. Data prediction reliability increases through standardization efforts combined with destructive correction of faulty data and amalgamation of multiple data sources. Additionally, researchers must be cautious of biases that may arise due to imbalanced datasets, such as overrepresentation of certain disease conditions or patient populations. Addressing these biases ensures that AI models generate equitable and effective therapeutic solutions.

To facilitate seamless collaboration and reproducibility in AI-driven drug discovery, adherence to Findable, Accessible, Interoperable, and Reusable (FAIR) data principles is crucial. These rules enable research teams and pharmaceutical enterprises to obtain high-quality training datasets for AI model development by providing transparent access to shared standardized information. The ability to find datasets easily becomes possible because of findability which involves proper documentation and indexing. The principle of accessibility allows data retrieval through proper guidelines. Interoperability allows different datasets to be integrated across various AI systems and research domains, while reusability ensures that data can be effectively utilized for future drug discovery projects. The implementation of FAIR principles fosters collaboration, accelerates innovation, and enhances the overall efficiency of AI-driven drug development [3].

AI has revolutionized drug discovery by leveraging data-driven approaches to optimize drug design, predict molecular interactions, and streamline clinical trials. The availability and quality of data are fundamental to the success of AI models, with structured and unstructured data playing complementary roles in enhancing predictive accuracy. An enhancement of AI-driven drug discovery dependability comes from using high-quality and unbiased datasets which follow rigorous validation and FAIR data principle requirements. The advancement of data collection and integration methods combined with management improvements will continue driving drug discovery through AI development for safer and more effective therapeutic medicine creation for medical conditions.

Types of Data in AI-Driven Drug Discovery

AI-driven drug discovery relies on vast and diverse datasets to enhance predictive modeling, optimize drug candidates, and improve the success rate of clinical trials. The integration of various data types allows AI models to simulate complex biological interactions, predict drug efficacy, and identify potential safety concerns. The data collection process contains five distinct sections which include chemical data and biological data and pharmacological data and clinical data and textual data. Each group serves fundamental purposes during the drug development phases [4].

Chemical Data

Chemical data forms the foundation of AI-driven drug discovery, as it enables the identification and optimization of novel drug candidates. This dataset primarily includes molecular structures, Simplified Molecular Input Line Entry System (SMILES) notation, and chemical fingerprints. The three-dimensional arrangements of drug molecules shown through molecular structures help AI models detect how these agents connect with biological targets. The text-based SMILES notation functions as a small and compact method to express molecular structure data in computational environments for simplified chemical data storage and processing purposes. The binary representations from chemical fingerprints enable researchers to perform similarity searches, execute virtual screening and accomplish compound clustering within AI-derived investigations. The data becomes essential for three main chemical functions: drug-likeness prediction, docking simulations, and molecular property estimation [5].

Biological Data

Biological data encompasses information about genes, proteins, cellular pathways, and metabolic networks that influence drug action. AI models analyze these datasets to identify potential drug targets and understand disease mechanisms. Genomic data includes DNA sequences and genetic variations that help predict individual responses to drugs, facilitating personalized medicine. AI algorithms derive information about protein structures and interactions alongside modifications through proteomic data to calculate drug-protein binding affinities. The evaluation of drug-induced gene regulation becomes possible through transcriptomic data that records gene expression profiles. Drug metabolic pathways can be understood through the study of small-molecule metabolites which make up metabolomic data. Integrating these datasets enables AI to simulate biological responses to drug candidates, improving target identification and validation (Figure 3.1).

Pharmacological Data

Pharmacological data is essential for evaluating drug safety and efficacy before clinical trials. This includes Absorption, Distribution, Metabolism, Excretion, and Toxicity (ADMET) profiles, which predict how a drug behaves in the human body. The effects of compounds on biological targets result in bioactivity assay findings that AI models use to determine drug candidate rankings. Pharmacological evaluation of drugs requires measurement of IC50 together with EC50 for determining potency along with therapeutic index. AI-driven pharmacokinetic models utilize these datasets to optimize drug formulations and dosing regimens, minimizing toxicity while maximizing therapeutic benefits [6].

Clinical Data

Clinical data plays a crucial role in AI-driven drug discovery by providing real-world insights into drug responses and patient outcomes. EHRs contain patient histories,

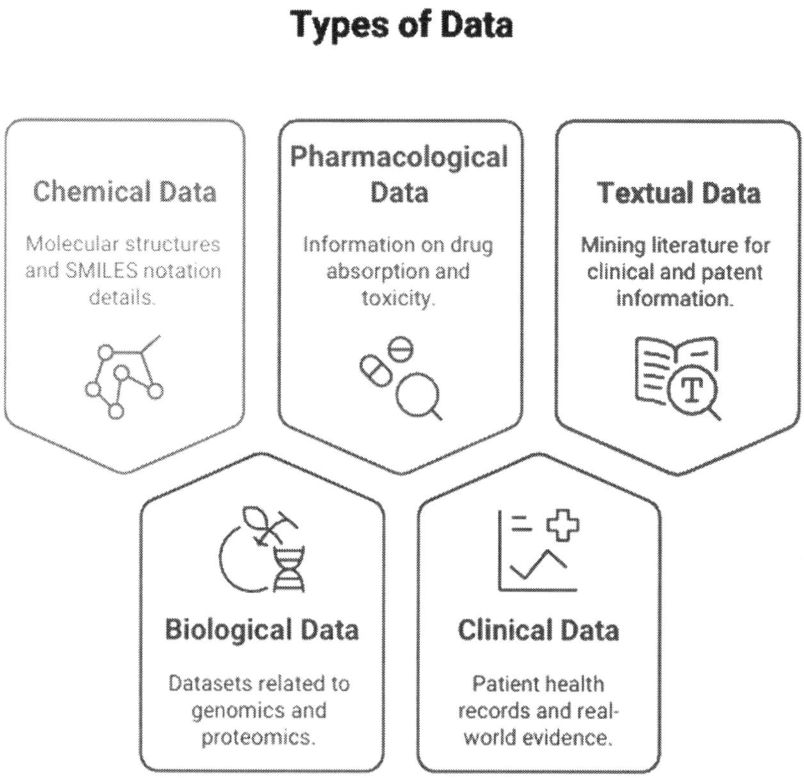

Figure 3.1 Types of Data

medication usage, and diagnostic reports, enabling AI models to identify biomarkers for disease progression and drug response. The validity of AI predictions for various patient groups depends on real-world evidence (RWE) which comprised observational studies and epidemiological data as well as post-market surveillance data. Through patient biomarker data obtained from diagnostic tests as well as genetic screenings precision medicine enables customized treatment methods according to each individual's genetic and physiological characteristics. The integration of clinical data with AI models enhances patient stratification, improves drug repurposing efforts, and accelerates the identification of novel therapeutic targets.

Textual Data

Textual data includes scientific literature, patents, and clinical trial reports, which contain vast amounts of valuable information for drug discovery. AI-driven literature mining from sources, such as PubMed, research articles, and conference proceedings, helps extract relationships between drugs, diseases, and targets. Analysis of patent registrations helps organizations identify both drug formulation advances and intellectual property (IP) status and estimate areas suitable for new pharmaceutical discoveries. The efficacy and safety profiles of drugs for various populations can be studied through reports of clinical trials available from FDA and ClinicalTrials.gov. NLP techniques enable AI to analyze and extract meaningful insights from these unstructured textual datasets, improving drug discovery predictions and decision-making [7].

Advanced Techniques in Data Collection

The rapid evolution of AI-driven drug discovery relies heavily on advanced data collection techniques that enhance the accuracy, depth, and applicability of datasets. Advanced screening systems along with single-cell sequencing and structural biology and real-world data (RWD) systems enable researchers to understand medical mechanisms and drug interactions and patients' response patterns completely. These sophisticated techniques ensure that AI models are trained on high-quality, representative data, leading to improved predictions and novel therapeutic discoveries [8].

High-Throughput Screening (HTS) and Data Integration

HTS is an essential technique in modern drug discovery, allowing researchers to test thousands to millions of compounds for potential biological activity against a specific target. The HTS platforms amalgamate automated robots and microfluidics systems which link to AI-based image detection processes for effective screening of big compound collections. AI algorithms merge and evaluate HTS data outputs to determine successful hit compounds while estimating secondary interactions during the lead selection process.

Additionally, data integration techniques merge HTS results with other datasets, such as genomics, proteomics, and cheminformatics, to provide a multi-dimensional view of drug-target interactions. The combined dataset feeds ML models that both enhance structure-activity relationship (SAR) understanding and speed up hit-to-lead optimization and improve predictive accuracy. The use of AI-powered multi-omics data fusion enables researchers to identify hidden data relationships that conventional analytic tools cannot detect leading to substantial connectivity rate increases during drug discovery processes [9].

Single-Cell Sequencing and Spatial Transcriptomics

Traditional bulk sequencing methods average gene expression across thousands of cells, potentially masking crucial variations in cellular behavior. Single-cell sequencing overcomes this limitation by enabling the analysis of gene expression at the level of individual cells, providing unprecedented insights into cell heterogeneity, disease progression, and drug responses. AI models use single-cell transcriptomics data for identifying cell subtypes and identifying disease specific biomarkers while determining drug resistance patterns.

Spatial transcriptomics goes a step further by preserving tissue architecture while capturing gene expression at the spatial level. This technique allows researchers to visualize how drugs affect different cell types within their native tissue environments. AI-based spatial analysis systems identify microscopic drug efficacy factors in environments which lead to product development of precise medicine strategies. Single-cell and spatial transcriptomics using DL processes generate high-resolution molecular maps that allow targeted drug development strategies [10].

Cryo-Electron Microscopy (Cryo-EM) and Structural Data Collection

Understanding drug-target interactions at the molecular level is critical for rational drug design. Cryo-EM has revolutionized structural biology by enabling the visualization of macromolecular complexes at near-atomic resolution. The method delivers three-dimensional data about proteins and nucleic acids together with understanding of ligand-binding characteristics which becomes vital in drug design that relies on protein structures.

AI-powered protein structure prediction algorithms, such as AlphaFold, leverage Cryo-EM, and crystallographic data to predict protein conformations with high accuracy. These AI models refine structural data by detecting dynamic protein-ligand interactions, optimizing lead compounds, and guiding fragment-based drug discovery. ML models enhance the speed of target validation and drug screening through automated analysis of Cryo-EM dataset output [11].

The integration of Cryo-EM with molecular docking simulations enhances drug discovery by enabling virtual screening of vast compound libraries against high-resolution protein structures. This method speeds up hit detection along with lead optimization campaigns while generating de novo drugs by lessening the need for high-end experimental tests.

Real-World Data (RWD) and Patient-Derived Models

RWD refers to patient health information collected outside of clinical trials, including EHRs, wearable device data, insurance claims, and patient registries. AI-driven models process this data to identify drug repurposing opportunities, real-time adverse effects, and treatment response patterns. AI uses NLP to extract valuable clinical information from unstructured text in medical records which makes post-market surveillance more effective and brings higher levels of precision medicine capabilities.

In addition to RWD, patient-derived models, such as organoids, patient-derived xenografts (PDXs), and induced pluripotent stem cells (iPSCs), provide a physiologically relevant system for drug screening. These models retain the genetic and epigenetic characteristics of the patient's disease, allowing AI-driven models to predict personalized treatment responses. Large patient-derived models feed data into ML algorithms for the purpose of developing superior drug combinations and prediction of resistance mechanisms and therapy optimization [12].

By integrating AI-powered analytics with RWD and patient-derived models, researchers can personalize drug development based on patient-specific molecular and clinical profiles. The method increases AI model prediction strength along with diminishing clinical trial failure and leads to the development of practical medications which demonstrate effectiveness.

Data Annotation and Curation Challenges in AI-Driven Drug Discovery

The success of AI in drug discovery is highly dependent on the quality, accuracy, and consistency of annotated data. Properly curated datasets enhance the predictive capabilities of AI models, enabling them to make more reliable predictions regarding drug efficacy, toxicity, and interactions. Data annotation and curation problems continue to act as a major barrier that reduces the total performance of AI systems in pharmaceutical research. The main barriers consist of standardization challenges and complex labeling of molecular bioactivity dependencies and dataset predisposition and intractable experimental data entry requirements. Addressing these challenges requires advanced computational approaches, automation, and collaboration among researchers, regulatory agencies, and pharmaceutical companies [13].

Standardization Issues in Chemical and Biological Databases

Drug discovery relies on vast amounts of chemical and biological data obtained from multiple sources, including public repositories, commercial databases, and proprietary pharmaceutical research. Each dataset presents various formatting inconsistencies as well as different ontology systems that limit data-sharing between platforms and platforms.

One of the critical challenges is the variation in molecular representations. Different cheminformatics platforms use multiple formats to depict the structure of chemical compounds. Two popular molecular notations, such as International Chemical Identifier (InChI) and SMILES, face data integration issues due to inconsistent representations that may cause mistakes during multi-source data combination. Similarly, differences in biological ontologies, such as Gene Ontology (GO), Medical Subject Headings (MeSH), and Disease Ontology (DO), make it difficult to align and compare datasets from various domains [14].

Another major concern is bioactivity data heterogeneity. Databases like ChEMBL, DrugBank, and PubChem store pharmacological data with different measurement units, experimental conditions, and scoring methods. For example, values, such as IC50, EC50, Ki, and Kd, indicate drug potency but can vary significantly depending on assay conditions and cell types used. AI systems need proper normalization to generate predictable results from unstandardized dataset training.

To mitigate these issues, researchers employ data standardization pipelines that harmonize diverse datasets into unified formats. Advanced algorithms, such as NLP-based entity recognition and ontology mapping, help resolve terminological inconsistencies. The implementation of FAIR data principles enables fully integrated platform interoperability by organizing datasets properly.

Labeling Challenges in Molecular Bioactivity Datasets

AI systems used for drug discovery need comprehensive and precise labeling regarding molecular bioactivity data. ML models need highly labeled datasets which contain clear information regarding drug-target binding and toxicity assessments as well as pharmacokinetic data and therapeutic effects parameters. However, the process of labeling molecular data is often complex and prone to errors [15].

One of the biggest challenges is the lack of ground truth data. Many pharmacological datasets rely on computational predictions rather than experimentally validated results. This introduces uncertainty, as predictions may not always reflect real biological interactions. The labeling process becomes problematic due to the existence of unclear or conflicting data tags. Researchers find that drugs generate various bioactivity patterns when they conduct their studies using diverse assay systems or biological test systems. The variations present in these datasets need proper management because they may confuse the Learning AI models.

Another limitation is the scarcity of labeled data for rare diseases and novel drug targets. AI models trained on common diseases with abundant data may struggle to make accurate predictions for orphan diseases with limited experimental data. Small datasets become usable for meaningful insight extraction through the combination of semi-supervised learning with self-supervised learning and few-shot learning techniques in research today. The label quality of datasets improves when experts utilize platforms like PubChem BioAssay and ChemBL together with crowdsourcing methods for annotation tasks [16].

Biases and Missing Values in Experimental Data

Bias in biomedical datasets is a major challenge that can lead to misleading AI predictions. Biases can arise from multiple sources, including dataset imbalance, experimental variability, and human annotation errors. Drug discovery datasets often present an unbalanced ratio between active compounds also known as positive results while inactive compounds or negative results occur infrequently. This imbalance can cause ML models to favor the majority class, leading to biased predictions that are not representative of real world scenarios.

Experimental variability further complicates AI-based predictions. Differences in assay conditions, instrument sensitivity, and cell line models introduce inconsistencies in experimental results. Different laboratories measure bioactivity values inconsistently because they implement varying concentrations of reagents and time exposure amounts as well as apply different data processing methodologies to the same compound. The inconsistent data used for training AI models creates barriers for effective finding generalization across different experimental conditions [17].

Additionally, missing values in datasets pose a significant problem. Many pharmacological datasets contain incomplete information due to experimental failures, limited availability of compounds, or restricted clinical data access. It is necessary to handle missing values correctly since ignoring them leads to incorrect predictions from AI models. Researchers employ data imputation techniques, such as multiple imputation by chained equations (MICE), k-nearest neighbors (KNN) imputation, and DL-based generative models, to estimate missing values and improve dataset completeness.

To address biases and missing data issues, researchers implement data augmentation strategies, adversarial training methods, and domain adaptation techniques. The approaches improve dataset diversity which enables better test-run generalization capabilities for AI models in realistic biomedical applications. Explainable AI (XAI) methods are also being integrated to identify and correct biased predictions, ensuring fairness and reliability in drug discovery applications.

Data Storage, Management, and Interoperability in AI-Driven Drug Discovery

In the field of AI-driven drug discovery, the ability to effectively store, manage, and integrate vast amounts of biomedical data is crucial. The complexity and diversity of datasets, ranging from chemical structures and biological sequences to pharmacokinetics and clinical records, require advanced storage solutions and standardized management practices. Efficient data handling enables AI models to process large amounts of data accurately which allows them to produce meaningful findings, thus speeding up drug discovery activities. To meet these demands, researchers rely on cloud computing platforms, standardized data-sharing principles like FAIR, and well-established ontologies and biomedical databases. These systems not only improve the efficiency of AI algorithms but also enhance collaboration and reproducibility in pharmaceutical research [18].

The evolution of cloud computing has revolutionized data storage and computational capabilities in drug discovery. Traditional local servers are often insufficient to handle the large-scale data generated by AI-driven research, necessitating scalable, high-performance solutions. Cloud platforms, such as Amazon Web Services (AWS), Google Cloud Platform (GCP), and Microsoft Azure, offer advanced storage and computational infrastructures that can process vast datasets in real time. The platforms offer instant access to computing power through which AI models can process big datasets effectively by eliminating the need for large-scale local hardware equipment. Furthermore, cloud-based solutions facilitate global collaboration, enabling researchers to securely share and access datasets from different institutions, fostering interdisciplinary advancements in drug discovery. Additionally, high-performance computing (HPC) environments integrated within these platforms, such as Tensor Processing Units (TPUs) and Graphics Processing Units (GPUs), accelerate the training of DL models for molecular property predictions, drug-target interactions, and toxicity assessments (Table 3.1).

To ensure that AI-driven drug discovery data is both reusable and reproducible, researchers adhere to the FAIR principles – Findability, Accessibility, Interoperability, and Reusability. These principles provide a structured approach to managing large-scale datasets, ensuring that data remains well-organized and easily

Table 3.1 Cloud Computing Platforms for AI-Driven Drug Discovery

Cloud Platform	*Key Features*	*Advantages*
Amazon Web Services (AWS)	Scalable storage, AI/ML tools (SageMaker), high-performance computing	Flexible, cost-effective, secure
Google Cloud Platform (GCP)	AI-powered analytics, BigQuery for large datasets, TPUs for AI acceleration	Fast processing, advanced AI integrations
Microsoft Azure	AI services, hybrid cloud support, strong compliance standards	Secure, enterprise-ready, scalable

retrievable for AI-driven analyses. The assignment of Digital Object Identifiers (DOIs) and PubChem Compound Identifiers (CIDs) and ChEMBL accession numbers establishes findability because researchers can easily identify specific datasets. Accessibility involves storing data in open-access repositories or cloud environments, allowing scientists worldwide to retrieve and utilize the information while adhering to privacy regulations [19]. Interoperability is critical for integrating heterogeneous datasets from multiple sources, requiring the use of standardized file formats, such as RDF, XML, and JSON, as well as metadata schemas that allow seamless data exchange between AI platforms. The Reusability principle makes possible effective dataset documentation accompanied by proper licensing so other researchers can verify initial results together with building new findings on established work. By following these principles, the pharmaceutical industry can maximize the utility of AI-driven drug discovery datasets, fostering transparency and innovation (Table 3.2).

A critical challenge in AI-based drug discovery is the harmonization of data from diverse sources, including chemical databases, genomic repositories, and clinical trial datasets. Ontologies and standardized biomedical databases play a fundamental role in ensuring that data from various fields is consistently labeled and structured. The GO functions as an ontology which creates specific classifications for biological functions along with molecular interactions and cellular pathways so AI models become effective at processing genomic and proteomic data. Similarly, the MeSH ontology standardizes terminology for biomedical literature, improving the efficiency of AI-driven literature mining for drug repurposing. Other essential

Table 3.2 FAIR Principles in Data Management

FAIR Principle	*Description*	*Examples*
Findable	Data should have unique identifiers and metadata	DOI, PubChem CID, ChEMBL ID
Accessible	Data should be easily retrievable via open-access platforms	Open-access repositories, cloud storage
Interoperable	Data should integrate with different systems and formats	XML, JSON, RDF for data exchange
Reusable	Data should be well-documented for future studies	Clear metadata, standardized licensing

ontologies include the DO, which maps relationships between diseases, genes, and potential therapeutic compounds, and the Chemical Entities of Biological Interest (ChEBI), which provides standardized annotations for chemical compounds [20].

In addition to ontologies, several well-established biomedical databases support AI-driven drug discovery. ChEMBL is a curated database containing bioactivity data for small molecules, including drug-target interactions and pharmacokinetics. AI model training heavily depends on PubChem because it contains comprehensive molecular structures alongside fingerprints and bioactivity test results. Kyoto Encyclopedia of Genes and Genomes (KEGG) provides widespread pathway analysis function that aids AI algorithms in drugs mechanism understanding as well as side effect prediction. DrugBank integrates chemical, pharmacological, and clinical data, supporting AI-based drug repurposing efforts by providing detailed insights into drug properties, molecular interactions, and approved indications. By leveraging these ontologies and databases, researchers can develop more precise and interpretable AI models that enhance drug discovery pipelines (Table 3.3).

Interoperability among diverse datasets is one of the most significant challenges in AI-driven drug discovery. Pharmaceutical research delivers different types of data through separate nomenclatures and units preventing systematic integration of study information from various projects. Standardization efforts, such as adopting machine-readable formats (JSON, XML) and implementing controlled vocabularies, help overcome these issues by ensuring that AI systems can seamlessly process and analyze different datasets. Moreover, the integration of Application Programming Interfaces (APIs) provided by databases like ChEMBL and DrugBank allows AI models to retrieve up-to-date information automatically, facilitating real-time data analysis and hypothesis generation [21].

The efficient storage, management, and interoperability of biomedical data are crucial for harnessing the full potential of AI in drug discovery. The combination between cloud computing environments that scale and perform well alongside FAIR principles enables proper organization of data for repeated use. Standardized

Table 3.3 Ontologies and Databases for AI-Driven Drug Discovery

Ontology/Database	*Purpose*	*Use in AI-Driven Drug Discovery*
Gene Ontology (GO)	Categorizes genes by function and cellular role	AI-driven target identification
MeSH (Medical Subject Headings)	Standardizes biomedical literature indexing	AI-powered literature mining
ChEMBL	Bioactivity data for small molecules	Virtual screening and drug repurposing
PubChem	Chemical structures, fingerprints, and bioactivity data	Molecular property prediction
KEGG	Pathway database for drug mechanisms	AI-assisted drug mechanism analysis
DrugBank	Chemical, pharmacological, and clinical drug data	Drug repurposing and toxicity analysis

Table 3.4 Interoperability Challenges and Solutions

Challenge	*Cause*	*Solution*
Diverse Data Formats	Different databases use different structures	Standardized formats like JSON, XML, RDF
Inconsistent Terminologies	Different names for the same molecules/genes	Use controlled vocabularies (MeSH, UniProt)
Limited Data Integration	Lack of real-time access to updated datasets	API-based integration (ChEMBL, DrugBank)

ontologies and biomedical databases play a key role in structuring and integrating diverse datasets, allowing AI models to extract meaningful insights for predicting drug efficacy, toxicity, and novel therapeutic targets. As the pharmaceutical industry continues to embrace AI-driven approaches, the development of robust data management frameworks will be essential in accelerating drug discovery and improving patient outcomes (Table 3.4).

AI-Powered Data Processing Pipelines in Drug Discovery

The integration of AI in drug discovery has significantly enhanced the efficiency and accuracy of data processing. By leveraging ML, DL, and Big Data analytics, AI enables researchers to analyze large datasets, predict molecular interactions, and optimize drug candidates more effectively. The AI pipelines reduce complex work processes that include drug-target interactions forecasting together with toxicity evaluations and structure-based medication and biomarker discovery. With the increasing availability of diverse biological and chemical data, AI-powered data pipelines play a pivotal role in accelerating the drug development process (Figure 3.2).

Machine Learning (ML) and Deep Learning (DL) Models

ML models are crucial for identifying patterns in complex biological and chemical datasets and making data-driven predictions. The drug discovery process depends on two primary sets of models called supervised and unsupervised learning which fulfill individual functions within drug discovery research [22].

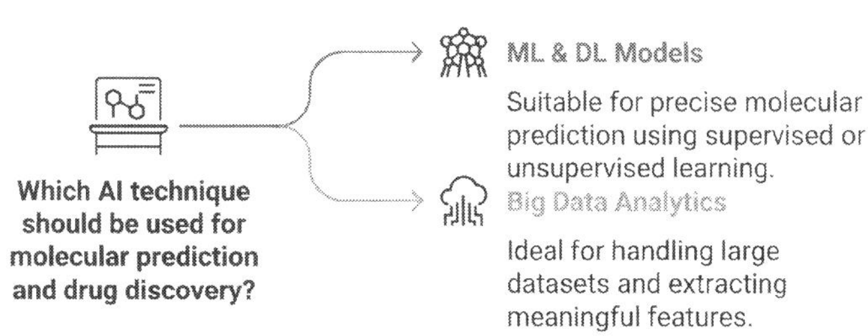

Figure 3.2 AI-Powered Data Processing Pipelines

In supervised learning, models are trained using labeled datasets where molecular properties or biological activities are already known. Algorithms, such as Random Forest (RF), Support Vector Machines (SVM), and Artificial Neural Networks (ANNs), are commonly employed to predict drug properties, including bioactivity levels (e.g., IC_{50} and EC_{50} values), solubility, and toxicity. These predictive frameworks for drug-likeness and pharmacokinetics develop through the analysis of molecular features that come from databases, including PubChem, ChEMBL, and DrugBank.

However, unsupervised learning is utilized for analyzing datasets without predefined labels. This approach is particularly useful for tasks, such as clustering compounds into chemical families, identifying novel drug scaffolds, and analyzing gene expression profiles. The research tools K-Means clustering and Hierarchical clustering and Principal Component Analysis (PCA) make it possible to organize similar molecule structures and discover previously invisible connections in extensive data collections. Dimensionality reduction techniques, such as t-Distributed Stochastic Neighbor Embedding (t-SNE) and Uniform Manifold Approximation and Projection (UMAP), are widely used for visualizing high-dimensional molecular data and understanding complex biological interactions [23].

A major breakthrough in AI-driven drug discovery is the development of transformer-based models that enhance molecular representation learning. Two leading DL predictive tools for protein structure prediction are AlphaFold alongside ChemBERTa and MolBERT. AlphaFold, developed by DeepMind, has revolutionized structural biology by providing near-experimental accuracy in protein 3D structure prediction, making it invaluable for drug-target interaction modeling and rational drug design. Similarly, ChemBERTa and MolBERT, inspired by NLP models, use self-attention mechanisms to analyze chemical representations, enabling improved predictions for drug potency, solubility, and metabolism.

Drug discovery has achieved further progress through Graph Neural Networks (GNNs) which use graphical representations of chemical compounds to predict molecular properties. GNNs allow AI models to capture intricate molecular relationships, leading to enhanced SAR predictions and de novo drug design approaches.

Big Data Analytics for Drug Discovery

The massive influx of data from HTS, genomics, proteomics, and EHRs necessitates advanced data analytics techniques. Big Data analytics supported by AI technology is essential for identifying valuable molecular information while improving drug candidate selection through optimized predictions of molecular structures.

One of the key challenges in drug discovery is handling datasets with thousands of molecular descriptors, many of which may be irrelevant or redundant. The performance of ML models improves because the selection techniques RFE, Lasso Regression and Genetic Algorithms discover the most important molecular features.

Additionally, dimensionality reduction techniques play a vital role in simplifying high-dimensional datasets and enabling more efficient data visualization.

PCA is widely used for reducing feature redundancy while preserving essential molecular properties. Meanwhile, t-SNE and UMAP are employed for clustering compounds and visualizing relationships in chemical space. Drug repurposing analyses and chemical diversity investigation and lead compound clustering operations are all possible through these analytical methods [24].

A critical advancement in AI-driven drug discovery is AI-powered automated feature extraction, which eliminates the need for manual molecular descriptor selection. Traditional cheminformatics methods depend solely on standardized chemical descriptors, including Lipinski's Rule of Five along with molecular fingerprints for their analysis. However, DL models can learn directly from raw molecular representations (e.g., SMILES strings, molecular graphs, and protein sequences) without manual intervention, resulting in more accurate bioactivity predictions and improved hit-to-lead optimization.

The Future of AI-Driven Drug Discovery

As AI-driven pipelines continue to evolve, the integration of multi-omics data, RWE, and federated learning is expected to further enhance drug discovery efforts. The development of cloud computing methods in combination with distributed AI frameworks enables researchers to execute more efficient data analysis on large datasets through protected data storage and streamlined institutional data exchange. The incorporation of real-world patient data, EHRs, and biomarker-driven approaches will enable precision medicine strategies, allowing for personalized drug development and targeted therapies.

By leveraging AI-powered data processing pipelines, ML models, and Big Data analytics, the pharmaceutical industry can significantly reduce drug discovery timelines, minimize costs, and improve the success rates of clinical trials. Drug discovery through AI depends on operational collaboration between computational intelligence and experimental validation to create safer and more effective and targeted medicines for complex diseases [25].

AI Ethics and Data Security in Drug Discovery

The integration of AI in drug discovery presents transformative opportunities, but it also raises critical ethical and security concerns. Ensuring data privacy, fairness, and transparency is essential to maintaining public trust and regulatory compliance. The processing of AI models depends on the analysis of extensive biological, chemical and clinical data while they also operate with sensitive patient records. Without proper governance, issues, such as data breaches, algorithmic bias, and unethical data usage, can significantly impact drug development outcomes. Therefore, robust frameworks for ethical AI deployment, secure data handling, and responsible AI governance are crucial for advancing drug discovery while upholding ethical standards (Figure 3.3).

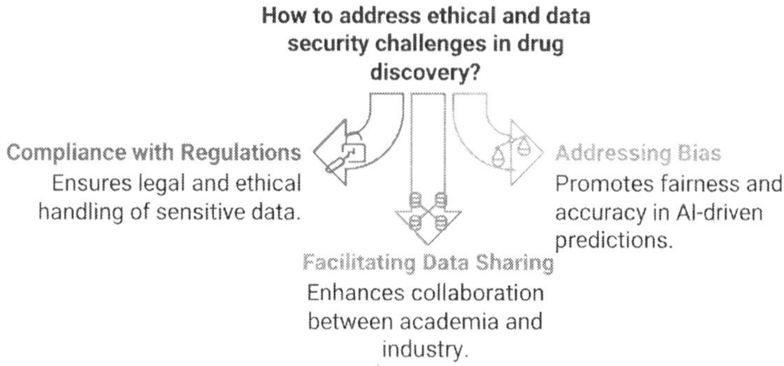

Figure 3.3 AI Ethics and Data Security

Handling Sensitive Patient Data under HIPAA/GDPR Compliance

The use of patient data in AI-driven drug discovery must adhere to strict legal and ethical regulations to prevent misuse and ensure privacy protection. Healthcare entities in the United States and European countries follow HIPAA and GDPR regulations which define how health information can be gathered and managed between healthcare providers [26].

Under HIPAA, organizations handling EHRs, genomic data, and real-world patient information must ensure data encryption, controlled access, and anonymization to prevent unauthorized use. The General Data Protection Regulation includes different data protection principles that incorporate both informed consent and the right to be forgotten and data minimization legislation. AI models trained on patient data must comply with these guidelines to ensure patient confidentiality and ethical research practices.

An important strategy to maintain privacy while utilizing valuable clinical data is the use of federated learning. With this method AI models acquire knowledge about medical data located throughout various healthcare institutions without divulging original medical records. By implementing privacy-preserving AI techniques, such as homomorphic encryption, differential privacy, and synthetic data generation, researchers can derive meaningful insights while safeguarding patient privacy [27].

Bias and Fairness in AI-Driven Predictions

AI models in drug discovery must be fair and unbiased to ensure that their predictions are reliable, equitable, and generalizable across diverse populations. The presence of bias in AI systems results from unbalanced training data and incomplete medical information as well as flawed experimental setups which causes incorrect medicine testing outcomes and disease biomarker errors and potentially unjust treatment distributions.

For example, an AI model trained primarily on Western population genetic data may fail to make accurate predictions for Asian or African populations, resulting in biased drug recommendations. Similarly, if an AI-driven drug screening system relies on historically biased datasets, it may overlook promising drug candidates or misinterpret toxicity profiles. Researchers need to tackle model biases through multiple steps, including adding various dataset samples alongside performing proper tests on fresh data and operating algorithms with built-in fairness optimization systems [28].

Moreover, AI models should be transparent and explainable, allowing researchers and regulators to understand how decisions are made. XAI methods, such as Shapley Additive Explanations (SHAP), Local Interpretable Model-Agnostic Explanations (LIME), and attention mechanisms in DL, can help interpret AI-driven predictions, ensuring accountability and regulatory approval.

Data-Sharing Challenges in Academia vs. Industry

Collaboration between academia, pharmaceutical companies, and regulatory agencies is essential for advancing AI-driven drug discovery. Challenges exist in data-sharing because organizations maintain hesitations about IP protection as well as commercial competition and patient data privacy guidelines.

In academia, open-access initiatives, such as Open Targets, ChEMBL, and PubChem, encourage data-sharing to accelerate research. Publicly available datasets enable AI models to learn from diverse biological and chemical data sources, facilitating drug repurposing, biomarker discovery, and novel target identification. Academic institutions work with limited processing capabilities along with restricted financial resources when handling wide datasets.

In contrast, the pharmaceutical industry maintains proprietary datasets that are not always accessible to the broader research community. Companies invest heavily in HTS, clinical trials, and compound libraries, making data-sharing challenging due to concerns over competitive advantage and regulatory constraints. Various data-sharing programs consisting of pre-competitive collaborations together with blockchain-based secure platforms and consortium research efforts help pharmaceutical firms establish safe and privacy-conscious data communication channels [29].

One promising approach to overcoming data-sharing barriers is the use of synthetic data – AI-generated datasets that mimic real patient or molecular data without exposing sensitive information. The implementation of artificial data enables AI model development and testing as well as regulatory inspections without risking the exposure of sensitive proprietary or private information.

Ensuring Ethical AI for the Future of Drug Discovery

As AI continues to revolutionize drug discovery, the need for robust ethical frameworks, transparent AI models, and secure data-sharing policies will become increasingly critical. Researchers must balance scientific progress with ethical responsibility, ensuring that AI-driven innovations benefit diverse patient populations, protect sensitive information, and promote fairness in drug development.

The pharmaceutical industry will fully harness the potential of AI when its leaders establish ethical principles and advanced security features in addition to responsible governance frameworks that protect against data misuse and privacy breaches and eliminate potential bias.

Future Trends in AI-Driven Data Management for Drug Discovery

As AI continues to revolutionize drug discovery, future advancements in data management and computational methodologies will play a crucial role in enhancing efficiency, accuracy, and scalability. Drastic changes in drug development pipelines are predicted through emerging technologies that include federated learning along with quantum computing and AI-driven hypothesis generation which provide better predictions and expedite drug repurposing while enhancing molecular simulations. The integration of these cutting-edge approaches will drive collaborative research, high-throughput drug screening, and novel therapeutic discoveries while maintaining data security and privacy [30].

Federated Learning for Multi-Center AI Drug Discovery Collaborations

Federated learning is an innovative approach that allows multiple research institutions, pharmaceutical companies, and hospitals to train AI models collaboratively without sharing raw data. Traditional AI models require data centralization, which raises privacy concerns and regulatory challenges, especially in clinical research. AI models utilizing federated learning function across decentralized datasets spread across several centers which helps maintain secure location of sensitive data.

In drug discovery, federated learning can be used for multi-site clinical trials, drug repurposing studies, and RWE analysis. Doctors and pharmaceutical entities can prepare AI models through diverse population training methods that stay compliant with privacy rules, such as HIPAA and GDPR. This decentralized approach enhances model generalization, ensuring that AI-driven predictions are more accurate, unbiased, and applicable to different populations [31].

Moreover, federated learning enables collaboration between academia and industry without compromising IP rights. Tailored implementations of secure aggregation techniques together with homomorphic encryption and differential privacy permit AI model training between institutions preserving the confidentiality of proprietary and confidential data. This fosters cross-border drug research, accelerates rare disease discoveries, and enhances AI-driven biomarker identification.

Quantum Computing for Molecular Simulations

Quantum computing is poised to redefine molecular simulations by exponentially improving the ability to model complex chemical interactions, protein folding, and drug-receptor binding dynamics. The computational complexity of classical methods makes it difficult to simulate complex biomolecular structures since modern processing limitations and high computational costs create significant barriers in accuracy. Quantum computing, however, leverages qubits and quantum entanglement to perform highly complex calculations in parallel, allowing for ultrafast molecular docking simulations and optimization of lead compounds.

One of the most significant applications of quantum computing in drug discovery is predicting molecular properties with higher precision. AI models together with quantum simulations deliver exact drug substance data which reduces wet-lab experimental requirements and their associated costs and durations. Quantum-enhanced AI models are also expected to accelerate de novo drug design, optimizing molecular structures in real time and identifying novel therapeutic candidates for diseases with limited treatment options [32].

Furthermore, pharmaceutical companies are exploring quantum machine learning (QML) for optimizing multi-target drug interactions, predicting adverse drug reactions, and simulating biological pathways. The companies Google along with IBM and D-Wave create quantum algorithms which transform structure-based drug design through their ability to find next-generation precision medicine by enhancing both drug specificity and treatment effectiveness.

AI-Powered Automated Hypothesis Generation in Drug Repurposing

AI is transforming drug repurposing by automating hypothesis generation, enabling rapid identification of existing drugs with potential new therapeutic applications. Traditional drug repurposing relies on manual literature reviews, clinical trial observations, and serendipitous discoveries. Complex biomedical datasets which contain EHRs and omics data along with scientific literature become accessible through systematic assessment by AI-driven analysis approaches.

One of the most promising AI-driven approaches is the use of knowledge graphs to identify novel drug candidates. Knowledge graphs integrate biological networks, protein interactions, metabolic pathways, and disease ontologies to map complex relationships between drugs, genes, and diseases. AI models examine pertinent relationships between drugs and diseases before generating hypotheses for established medicine utilization as treatment of different health conditions. For example, AI-powered platforms have successfully identified existing antiviral and anti-inflammatory drugs as potential treatments for emerging infectious diseases like COVID-19 [33].

Additionally, NLP and DL models are being used to mine biomedical literature and patents, identifying previously overlooked drug interactions. Data mining through NLP enables IBM Watson for Drug Discovery and BenevolentAI to search through millions of studies for findings which guide researchers toward new drug potential.

By integrating AI with RWE, researchers can validate hypothesis-driven drug repurposing strategies using patient health records, adverse event reports, and clinical trial data. A drug repurposing approach benefits medical needs by cutting development times while decreasing expenses and raising the likelihood of success to provide patients with rapid access to repurposed medicines [34].

References

1. Wouters, O. J., McKee, M., & Luyten, J. (2020). Estimated research and development investment needed to bring a new medicine to market, 2009–2018. *JAMA*, *323*(9), 844–853.
2. Paul, S. M., Mytelka, D. S., Dunwiddie, C. T., Persinger, C. C., Munos, B. H., Lindborg, S. R., & Schacht, A. L. (2010). How to improve R&D productivity: The pharmaceutical industry's grand challenge. *Nature Reviews Drug Discovery*, *9*(3), 203–214.
3. Aminabee, S. K., Prabhakar, M. C., Prasad, R. G. S. V., & Lakshmana Rao, A. (2011). Screening the pharmacological activity of cerium oxide nanoparticles in-vitro. *Biomedical and Pharmacology Journal*, *4*(2), 287–289.
4. Murmu, A., & Gyorffy, B. (2024). Artificial intelligence methods available for cancer research. *Frontiers in Medicine*, *18*, 778–797.
5. Ocaña, A., Pandiella, A., Siu, L. L., & Tannock, I. F. (2011). Preclinical development of molecular-targeted agents for cancer. *Nature Reviews Clinical Oncology*, *8*(4), 200–209.
6. Amir, E., Seruga, B., Martinez-Lopez, J., & Ocana, A. (2011). Oncogenic targets, magnitude of benefit, and market pricing of antineoplastic drugs. *Journal of Clinical Oncology*, *29*(18), 2543–2549.
7. Aminabee, S. K., Lakshmana Rao, A., Sowmya, K., Nymisha, D., Kusuma Naga Lakshmi, K., Manikanta, K. V. N. S., & Praveen Kumar, P. (2019). Evaluation of analgesic activity of *Ficus palmata*. *Iranian Journal of Pharmaceutical Sciences*, *15*(3), 47–60.
8. Chang, L., Lee, Y., Kim, H., & Sellers, W. R. (2023). Systematic profiling of conditional pathway activation identifies context-dependent synthetic lethalities. *Nature Genetics*, *55*, 1709–1720.
9. Vazquez, F., & Sellers, W. R. (2021). Are CRISPR screens providing the next generation of therapeutic targets? *Cancer Research*, *81*(22), 5806–5809.
10. Aminabee, S. K., Lakshmana Rao, A., & Chinna Eswaraiah, M. (2020). In-vivo antioxidant activity of different fractions of *Indigofera barberi* against paracetamol-induced toxicity in rats. *Turkish Journal of Pharmaceutical Sciences*, *17*(2), 136–140.
11. Wang, T., Birsoy, K., Hughes, N. W., Krupczak, K. M., Post, Y., Wei, J. J., & Sabatini, D. M. (2015). Identification and characterization of essential genes in the human genome. *Science*, *350*(6264), 1096–1101.
12. Tiedt, R., et al. (2023). Integrated CRISPR screening and drug profiling identifies combination opportunities for EGFR, ALK, and BRAF/MEK inhibitors. *Cell Reports*, *42*(1), 112003.
13. Prasanth, D. S. N. B. K., Aminabee, S. K., Lakshmana Rao, A., Teja, N., Bhargavi, K., Monika, C., Pujitha, B., Sandhya, T., Lalitha, A., & Siva Prasad, P. (2020). Anthelmintic activity of *Mansoa alliacea* against *Pheretima posthuma*: In-vitro and in-silico approach. *Thai Journal of Pharmaceutical Sciences*, *4*(3), 186–196.
14. Sulahian, R., et al. (2019). Synthetic lethal interaction of SHOC2 depletion with MEK inhibition in RAS-driven cancers. *Cell Reports*, *29*(5), 118–134.e8.
15. Kryukov, G. V., et al. (2016). MTAP deletion confers enhanced dependency on the PRMT5 arginine methyltransferase in cancer cells. *Science*, *351*(6278), 1214–1218.
16. Prasanth, D. S. N. B. K., Aminabee, S. K., Lakshmana Rao, A., Guntupalli, C., Reddy, A. R., Kulandaivelu, U., Rao, S. N. K., & Rajeshwari, P. (2021). Inhibitory effects of *Mansoa alliacea* in Freund's adjuvant arthritis on inflammatory markers and its confirmation by in-silico strategy. *Thai Journal of Pharmaceutical Sciences*, *45*(6), 532–544.
17. Rask-Andersen, M., Almen, M. S., & Schioth, H. B. (2011). Trends in the exploitation of novel drug targets. *Nature Reviews Drug Discovery*, *10*(8), 579–590.
18. Imming, P., Sinning, C., & Meyer, A. (2006). Drugs, their targets and the nature and number of drug targets. *Nature Reviews Drug Discovery*, *5*(10), 821–834.
19. Hopkins, A. L., & Groom, C. R. (2002). The druggable genome. *Nature Reviews Drug Discovery*, *1*(9), 727–730.

20. Aminabee, S. K., Santhi Krupa, D., Hanumanth Rao, K., Sirisha, V., Anitha Kumari, V., Nagasen, D., Sujiya, B., & Leelavati, T. S. (2023). Pharmacoeconomic analysis of biologic vs. biosimilar therapies in rheumatoid arthritis. *International Journal of Chemical and Biochemical Sciences*, *24*(4), 395–400.
21. Arkin, M. R., & Wells, J. A. (2004). Small-molecule inhibitors of protein-protein interactions: Progressing towards the dream. *Nature Reviews Drug Discovery*, *3*(4), 301–317.
22. Nevola, L., & Giralt, E. (2015). Modulating protein–protein interactions: The potential of peptides. *Chemical Communications*, *51*(16), 3302–3315.
23. Leelavati, T. S., Madhavi, S., Kamal, G., Raju, P. V. M., Susmitha, K., Vinod, M., & Aminabee, S. K. (2023). Revolutionizing healthcare delivery: Telemedicine's influence on access and patient satisfaction. *International Journal of Chemical and Biochemical Sciences*, *24*(5), 106–115.
24. Macarron, R., Banks, M. N., Bojanic, D., Burns, D. J., Cirovic, D. A., Garyantes, T., & Hertzberg, R. P. (2011). Impact of high-throughput screening in biomedical research. *Nature Reviews Drug Discovery*, *10*(3), 188–195.
25. Liew, S. K., Malagobadan, S., Arshad, N. M., & Nagoor, N. H. (2020). A review of the structure–activity relationship of natural and synthetic antimetastatic compounds. *Biomolecules*, *10*(1), 138.
26. Aminabee, S. K., Devi Mallika, K., & Lakshmana Rao, A. (2023). Natural resources in management and treatment of diseases: A review. *Pharma Times*, *55*(11), 7–10.
27. Benitez, J. C., et al. (2021). Late phase 1 studies: Concepts and outcomes. *The Lancet Oncology*, *22*(10), e446–e455.
28. Eisenhauer, E. A., O'Dwyer, P. J., Christian, M., & Humphrey, J. S. (2000). Phase I clinical trial design in cancer drug development. *Journal of Clinical Oncology*, *18*(3), 684–692.
29. Aminabee, S. K., & Lakshmana Rao, A. (2024). Computational identification of selected bioactive compounds from *Cedrus deodara* as inhibitors against SARS-CoV-2 main protease: A pharmacoinformatics study. *Indian Drugs*, *61*(2), 78–91.
30. Chan, H. C. S., Shan, H., Dahoun, T., Vogel, H., & Yuan, S. (2019). Advancing drug discovery via artificial intelligence. *Trends in Pharmacological Sciences*, *40*(8), 592–604.
31. Chang, L., Ruiz, P., Ito, T., & Sellers, W. R. (2021). Targeting pan-essential genes in cancer: Challenges and opportunities. *Cancer Cell*, *39*(4), 466–479.
32. Rudolph, J., Settleman, J., & Malek, S. (2021). Emerging trends in cancer drug discovery from drugging the undruggable to overcoming resistance. *Cancer Discovery*, *11*(4), 815–821.
33. Ravi Shankar, K., Aminabee, S. K., Ramana, G., Chenchu Lakshmi, K. N. V., & Indusree, G. (2024). Formulation and evaluation of propranolol hydrochloride floating tablets by 32 factorial design. *International Journal of Drug Delivery Technology*, *14*(4), 2060–2067.
34. Menyhart, O., & Gyorffy, B. (2021). Multi-omics approaches in cancer research with applications in tumor subtyping, prognosis, and diagnosis. *Computational and Structural Biotechnology Journal*, *19*, 949–960.

4 AI-Driven Drug Target Identification

Introduction to AI in Drug Target Identification

The process of drug target identification has traditionally relied on experimental methods, such as high-throughput screening (HTS), biochemical assays, and functional genomics. Best practices in therapeutic target discovery exist but encounter various performance problems along with expensive operations and lengthy validation procedures. Artificial Intelligence (AI) introduced drug discovery to new modern methods which transform research by allowing scientists to use predictive and systematic and data-driven methodologies instead of traditional practice. The combination of biological datasets and computational models and machine learning (ML) algorithms allows AI systems to speed up and precisely identify and validate potential drug targets. By integrating AI into drug discovery pipelines, researchers can prioritize targets based on disease relevance, molecular interactions, and predictive modeling, ultimately accelerating the development of novel therapeutics [1].

One of the key advantages of AI in target identification is its ability to analyze complex biological networks and discover previously unknown relationships between genes, proteins, and disease phenotypes. Through deep learning (DL) and graph-based algorithm processing of biological data records AI models achieve better drug target identification performance than traditional pharmacological techniques. AI models assess comprehensive genomic information in combination with transcriptomic information and proteomic information and metabolomic information in order to discover new biomarkers and estimate drug substance relationships while enhancing the effectiveness of potential candidate drugs [2]. By automating the target selection and validation process, AI minimizes the reliance on trial-and-error experimentation, significantly reducing the cost and time required for drug development.

The integration of multi-omics and large-scale biological datasets plays a critical role in AI-driven target identification. Multiple biological scales become accessible through analysis of multi-omics data that spans genomic and transcriptomic and proteomic and metabolomic information. Integrating various datasets with AI analytics methods enables detection of hidden patterns which traditional analysis methods would otherwise miss. AI examines genotypic disease-related changes to

DOI: 10.4324/9781003616177-4

forecast protein functional modifications that could become suitable drug targets. Additionally, AI algorithms can process real-world biological datasets, such as electronic health records (EHRs), clinical trial reports, and patient biomarker data, to identify personalized therapeutic targets for precision medicine [3].

The functionality of biomolecular targets for drug development benefits from AI predictions which determine the effects of selecting different biomolecular targets. Existing drug-target interaction databases become accessible to ML models that would enable them to identify high-confidence targets and propose alternative therapeutic pathways. AI-based tools, such as DL models, natural language processing (NLP) systems for literature mining, and knowledge graphs for systems biology, further aid in uncovering potential drug targets. Computational methods optimize drug discovery operations by conducting quick large-scale biochemical interaction assessments that show the most effective therapeutic directions [4].

AI is revolutionizing drug target identification by introducing automation, predictive analytics, and deep biological insights into the discovery process. AI allows researchers to use DL models for quick and accurate identification of drug targets through multi-omics data analysis and large-scale biological dataset analysis. The new approach collates drug development at a faster rate and delivers precision medicine through medications that consider unique patient information. As AI technology continues to advance, its role in drug discovery will expand, offering new opportunities for developing highly targeted and effective treatments for various diseases [5].

Computational Approaches for Target Identification

Machine Learning (ML) and Deep Learning (DL) Models

The combination of ML and DL technologies strengthen drug target identification through predictive analytics and automation features along with large-scale data processing capabilities. The application of ML models in drug discovery happens via supervised and unsupervised learning methods. In supervised learning, algorithms are trained on labeled datasets where known drug-target interactions or disease-associated genes serve as ground truth. These models can predict novel drug-target interactions, classify disease-related genes, and prioritize targets based on their therapeutic relevance. Unsupervised learning techniques uncover unknown relationships by detecting hidden patterns in biological data which lacks pre-existing labels while identifying clusters in the data. The identification of new therapeutic opportunities depends heavily on clustering methods along with dimensionality reduction and anomaly detection methods [6].

A major breakthrough in AI-driven drug discovery is the emergence of transformer-based architectures. Models like AlphaFold, developed by DeepMind, use DL to predict protein structures with near-experimental accuracy, facilitating the identification of potential drug-binding sites. The Graph Networks developed by DeepMind combine with AI models, such as ChemBERTa, MolBERT along with ESMFold to examine molecular bonds and forecast target characteristics, which

Table 4.1 Machine Learning (ML) and Deep Learning (DL) Models in Target Discovery

ML/DL Approach	*Description*	*Application in Target Discovery*
Supervised Learning	Uses labeled datasets to train models to predict target properties.	Predicting drug-target interactions, classifying disease-associated genes.
Unsupervised Learning	Finds hidden patterns in unlabeled data.	Clustering similar drug targets, discovering novel biological pathways.
Transformer-Based Models	Uses attention mechanisms to model biological sequences.	Protein folding prediction (AlphaFold), molecular interaction prediction (DeepMind's Graph Networks).

helps in designing drugs rationally. These advanced architectures allow for rapid screening of millions of potential drug-target interactions, significantly reducing the time required for target validation and accelerating the transition from discovery to preclinical testing (Table 4.1).

Graph Neural Networks (GNNs) in Target Identification

The rise of GNNs has proven to be an efficient computational system which executes excellent drug-target interaction predictions and disease-associated protein identification. GNNs differ from typical tabular ML models because they process biological networks, such as PPI networks together with gene regulatory networks and metabolic pathways. By representing biological data as graphs, GNNs learn the relationships between nodes (e.g., proteins, genes, and small molecules) and edges (e.g., interactions and binding affinities), allowing them to predict novel therapeutic targets with high confidence [7].

One of the key applications of GNNs in drug target identification is the prediction of protein-protein interactions. Through pathway analysis researchers can locate proteins which demonstrate possible drug accessibility. Using AI tools GNNs process extensive PPI datasets along with functional module identification to select targets for disease relevance using network topology and centrality analysis. Additionally, these models facilitate network-based drug repurposing by mapping known drugs onto disease-specific interaction networks, uncovering alternative therapeutic applications for existing drugs [8].

GNNs establish a vital function for network-based priority determination of disease-related targets. The existing process of target selection depends on both screening large datasets and conducting experimental tests which proves to be both expensive in cost and time-consuming. The algorithmical process becomes faster through GNNs because these networks combine various omics datasets to accurately identify target-disease relationships. By leveraging large-scale genomic and transcriptomic data, AI-powered GNNs can identify novel biomarkers, refine drug target predictions, and optimize lead compounds for precision medicine (Table 4.2).

Table 4.2 Graph Neural Networks (GNNs) in Target Identification

GNN Approach	*Function*	*Application in Drug Discovery*
Predicting Protein-Protein Interactions	Models protein-protein interaction networks.	Identifies disease-relevant protein targets.
Drug-Target Interaction Prediction	Uses graph-based features to analyze molecular structures.	Predicts potential drug candidates for specific targets.
Network-Based Target Prioritization	Ranks disease-associated genes and proteins.	Helps prioritize novel therapeutic targets.

Natural Language Processing (NLP) for Target Discovery

NLP through its innovation allows researchers to retrieve beneficial insights directly from scientific documents and clinical trial records as well as patent databases. The AI-powered NLP models PubMedBERT, BioBERT along with SciBERT facilitate the automatic extraction of drug target information from literature bases. These models analyze vast repositories of biomedical publications, extracting relevant information about disease mechanisms, gene-disease associations, and novel therapeutic targets [9]. By scanning millions of research articles, NLP-driven AI can highlight promising candidates for experimental validation, significantly reducing the time required for hypothesis generation.

The NLP-powered systems extract critical insights from ClinicalTrials.gov and the European Medicines Agency (EMA) databases which are accessible publicly. NLP models analyze court reports to detect beneficial medical treatments while predicting new drugs delivered from existing medications. AI-driven NLP also plays a role in analyzing patent landscapes, helping researchers assess intellectual property trends, identify emerging drug targets, and optimize drug development strategies [10].

The combination of NLP techniques recognizes early drug effects and toxicities by applying sentiment analysis on patient records alongside topic modeling of EHRs and adverse event reports. AI-powered text mining tools can extract meaningful associations between genetic variations and disease phenotypes, contributing to precision medicine approaches and patient-specific treatment strategies (Table 4.3).

Table 4.3 Natural Language Processing (NLP) for Target Discovery

NLP Approach	*Function*	*Application in Drug Discovery*
Literature Mining (PubMedBERT)	Extracts key findings from scientific literature.	Identifies new drug targets from PubMed, patents, and clinical trial reports.
AI-Driven Insights from Clinical Trials	Analyzes trial data for potential target molecules.	Predicts emerging drug targets and repurposing opportunities.

Omics-Driven AI Target Discovery

The combination of AI and multi-omics data brought dramatic advances to the discovery of targets for new drugs during development. Systems biology and genomics alongside proteomics along with metabolomics allow AI models to analyze extensive biological data for identifying precise novel drug targets. AI-driven analytics enable the identification of disease-associated genes, predict protein-ligand interactions, and uncover metabolic pathways crucial for therapeutic interventions [11]. The synergy between AI and omics technologies accelerates the drug discovery process, enhances precision medicine, and facilitates the identification of previously unexplored therapeutic targets (Figure 4.1).

Genomics and AI-Based Target Prioritization

Genomic data plays essential functions in drug target discoveries because it reveals genetic patterns that help understand disease risks and detect disease markers. Computer systems using GWAS technology now enable researchers to analyze vast genomic resources through which they discover genetic features associated with diseases. Traditional GWAS approaches require extensive statistical analyses, but AI models, particularly DL architectures, enhance the predictive power of these studies by identifying non-linear associations and complex interactions within genomic data. AI-driven GWAS can prioritize disease-associated genes, refine genetic risk scores, and facilitate target selection for personalized medicine [12].

CRISPR-based functional genomics screens provide another powerful tool for identifying essential genes involved in disease mechanisms. The implementation of AI models in CRISPR screening involves data analysis of extensive knockout collections along with genomic score prediction and molecular interaction-combined phenotypic observation result interpretation. ML algorithms processing CRISPR screening data enable the identification of therapeutic genes that speeds up drug discovery activities. AI-powered integration of CRISPR and GWAS datasets further improves the identification of actionable genetic targets, allowing for a more refined approach to precision medicine [13].

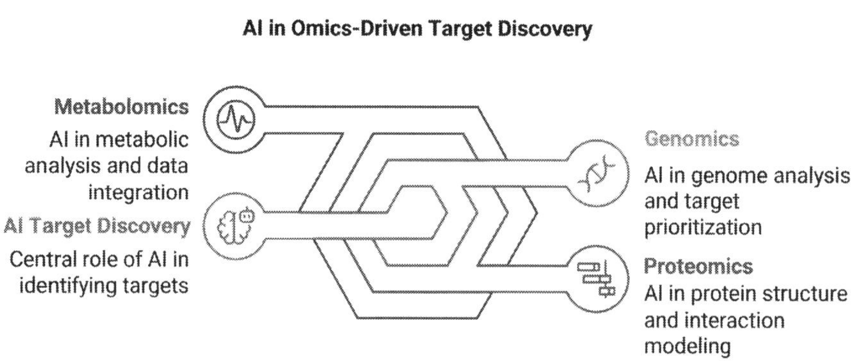

Figure 4.1 AI in Omics-Driven Target Discovery

Proteomics and Structural Biology

Proteomics, the large-scale study of proteins and their interactions, plays a crucial role in drug target discovery. AI technologies have reached a new milestone through AlphaFold because this model uses sophisticated algorithms to achieve laboratory-grade precision in protein folding predictions. This breakthrough allows researchers to explore previously undetermined protein structures, facilitating the identification of novel druggable targets. AI-based structural biology expedites our comprehension of protein movements alongside enzymatic alterations along with protein-binding interactions because these knowledge points direct therapeutic development processes [14].

In addition to structural prediction, AI is used for protein-ligand interaction modeling, a key aspect of rational drug design. High-throughput docking simulations undergo DL model analysis for binding affinity detection while the models enhance ligand optimization procedures. AI through DeepDock and AtomNet relies on convolutional neural networks (CNNs) and reinforcement learning to identify superior compounds matching specific targets through their molecular docking algorithms. The methods shorten experimental testing requirements because they decrease the resources needed and accelerate medication discovery protocols [15].

Furthermore, AI-enhanced mass spectrometry and proteomic profiling allow for the identification of disease biomarkers, post-translational modifications, and novel protein targets. AI models analyze big proteomics data, while they recognize disease-specific protein characteristics and establish links between these features and pharmaceutical results. The advancement allows scientists to develop AI-based precision medicine practices which prescribe individualized treatments according to proteomic data.

Metabolomics and Systems Biology Approaches

Metabolomics, the study of small-molecule metabolites in biological systems, provides a comprehensive view of cellular processes, making it a valuable tool in drug target identification. AI systems through metabolic pathway evaluation enable scientists to discover essential enzymes and metabolites which guide disease development. AI models connect multi-omics data, such as transcriptome information and metabolomics information to find new treatment targets along with detecting disease-related metabolic weaknesses [16].

Systems biology approaches leverage AI to construct and analyze complex biological networks, such as metabolic and signaling pathways. AI-driven network analysis helps map interactions between genes, proteins, and metabolites, providing a holistic understanding of disease mechanisms. Using this network-level examination scientists gain the ability to find treatment targets among these network elements which can become specific drug targets. The AI-driven metabolic analysis tools FBA and COBRA help determine how metabolic fluxes evolve when drugs are introduced by assessing altered drug responses to guide drug reutilization plans [17].

By integrating metabolomics with AI, researchers can identify metabolic biomarkers, predict drug responses, and optimize therapeutic strategies. AI software performs crucial metabolic pathway examinations during oncology studies because cancer cells demonstrate novel metabolic reaction depending patterns. Laboratory data from tumor metabolomics allows the development of precision therapies by helping machines determine cancer metabolic vulnerabilities.

AI-Driven Network Pharmacology and Multi-Target Drug Discovery

Target-Disease Network Mapping Using AI

Network pharmacology integrates systems biology with pharmacology to understand complex drug-target interactions across multiple biological networks. This domain has received a revolutionary transformation from AI through its abilities to analyze diseases on a large scale and discover new therapeutic possibilities. Tremendous biological datasets feed AI algorithms which utilize disease-specific interaction networks for identifying important molecular elements that drive pathogenesis. These networks integrate genomic, proteomic, metabolomic, and transcriptomic data to identify critical nodes – genes, proteins, or metabolites that could serve as potential drug targets [18].

The application of AI-based structural biology improves scientists' comprehension of proteins' structural transitions and modifications and their interactions with other proteins that prove crucial for pharmaceutical development. ML and DL models can predict how specific genetic mutations influence disease progression by analyzing large-scale patient datasets, allowing researchers to pinpoint potential therapeutic interventions. Through DL models scientists evaluate many docking simulations to estimate binding relationships while enhancing ligand optimization. ML algorithms in DeepDock and AtomNet predict optimal compounds for specific protein targets through the combination of CNNs and reinforcement learning. The methods shorten experimental testing requirements because they decrease the resources needed and accelerate medication discovery protocols [19].

Polypharmacology and Multi-Target Drug Design

Traditional drug discovery has focused on the "one drug, one target" approach. However, many complex diseases, such as cancer, neurodegenerative disorders, and metabolic syndromes, involve multiple molecular pathways, making single-target therapies less effective. Computer models analyze extensive proteomics datasets to recognize disease-capturing protein patterns then link those patterns to specific treatments through analysis. The advanced developments enable medical practitioners to deliver precision medicine treatments which are optimized for each patient's proteomic information [20].

AI is also transforming the prediction of off-target effects – an essential aspect of drug safety. While conventional computational approaches often miss hidden drug interactions, DL models trained on large pharmacological databases can predict potential side effects by analyzing molecular similarity patterns. A metabolic pathway model created by AI methodology reveals what regulatory enzymes and disease-specific metabolites mostly affect disease progression. AI models unify metabolomics together with transcriptomics data collected from various datasets to discover new treatment targets alongside disease state metabolic weakness predictions [21].

Another breakthrough in AI-driven drug discovery is drug repurposing, where existing drugs are computationally screened for new therapeutic indications. Using this network-level examination scientists gain the ability to find treatment targets among these network elements which can become specific drug targets. The combination of FBA and COBRA along with AI-based analysis provides mathematical tools to forecast metabolic flux alterations from drug manifestation which directs medical researchers toward drug rediscovery targets.

Additionally, AI is enhancing synergistic drug combination discovery, a crucial aspect of multi-target therapy. AI software performs crucial metabolic pathway examinations during oncology studies because cancer cells demonstrate novel metabolic reaction depending patterns. Tumor metabolomics data processed by ML models enables researchers to discover metabolic weaknesses which lead to the development of selective cancer-targeted therapy approaches. Moreover, AI-assisted screening of approved drug combinations allows researchers to identify novel synergistic pairs that may provide superior therapeutic benefits compared to single-agent treatments [22].

AI introduces large-scale computational analysis methods that investigate disease-related pathways for predicting newly potential therapeutic targets. AI algorithms analyze extensive biological datasets to generate disease-specific network models which identify essential molecular players that contribute to disease development. The ability of AI to process and analyze large-scale biological networks, predict drug interactions, and optimize therapeutic strategies is transforming modern pharmacology, paving the way for more precise and personalized medicine (Table 4.4).

AI Powered Virtual Screening for Target Validation

Computerized drug discovery underwent a transformation through virtual screening because it delivers fast target identification paired with validated potential drug candidates. The process of virtual screening becomes more effective and precise through AI methods which integrate DL algorithms combined with ML and enhanced molecular modeling approaches. AI-based virtual screening technology can decrease time and expenses in experimental screening while speeding up drug discovery workflows [23].

AI-Based Molecular Docking and Binding Affinity Predictions

Molecular docking is a crucial step in structure-based drug discovery, as it predicts the interaction between small molecules and biological targets. Traditional docking approaches rely on physics-based scoring functions to estimate binding affinity; however, AI has introduced ML-based scoring functions that significantly

Table 4.4 AI-Driven Approaches in Network Pharmacology and Multi-Target Drug Discovery

Aspect	*Description*	*AI Techniques Used*
Target-Disease Network Mapping	AI-driven identification of disease-associated molecular pathways by integrating multi-omics data (genomics, proteomics, metabolomics).	Graph Neural Networks (GNNs), Machine Learning (ML), Deep Learning (DL)
Pathway Enrichment Analysis	AI analyzes omics data to highlight critical pathways involved in disease progression, uncovering novel drug targets.	Supervised Learning, Unsupervised Learning, Network-Based AI Models
Polypharmacology and Multi-Target Drug Design	AI predicts interactions of drugs with multiple disease-related proteins, leading to more effective therapies.	Deep Learning, Molecular Docking AI, Virtual Screening Algorithms
Off-Target Effects Prediction	AI predicts unintended drug interactions to improve drug safety and reduce side effects.	Reinforcement Learning, Multitask Learning, Large-Scale Pharmacological Databases
Drug Repurposing	AI identifies new therapeutic uses for existing drugs, reducing development time and costs.	Natural Language Processing (NLP), AI-Driven Knowledge Graphs, Transfer Learning
Synergistic Drug Combinations	AI analyzes drug interactions to identify synergistic effects, optimizing combination therapy.	Reinforcement Learning, AI-Enabled High-Throughput Screening, Predictive Modeling

improve the accuracy of these predictions. The training of ML models occurs through vast amounts of experimentally obtained ligand-receptor binding data which enables enhanced precision in predicting binding affinities [24].

AI also plays a key role in predicting small molecule-protein interactions by analyzing vast chemical and structural datasets. The protein structure prediction capabilities of AlphaFold and DeepMind's Graph Networks as transformer-based architectures lead to enhanced molecular docking predictions by offering atomic-level accuracy in protein structure predictions. Reinforcement learning algorithms now serve to find the best ligand conformations along with determining stable binding positions for target proteins.

In Silico High-Throughput Screening (HTS) Using AI

HTS is an essential step in drug discovery, enabling the rapid screening of large chemical libraries for potential drug candidates. AI-driven in silico HTS enhances this process by using generative models and DL techniques to predict drug-target interactions on a large scale. The deep generative models VAEs and GANs create new molecular structures which possess drug-like characteristics through their

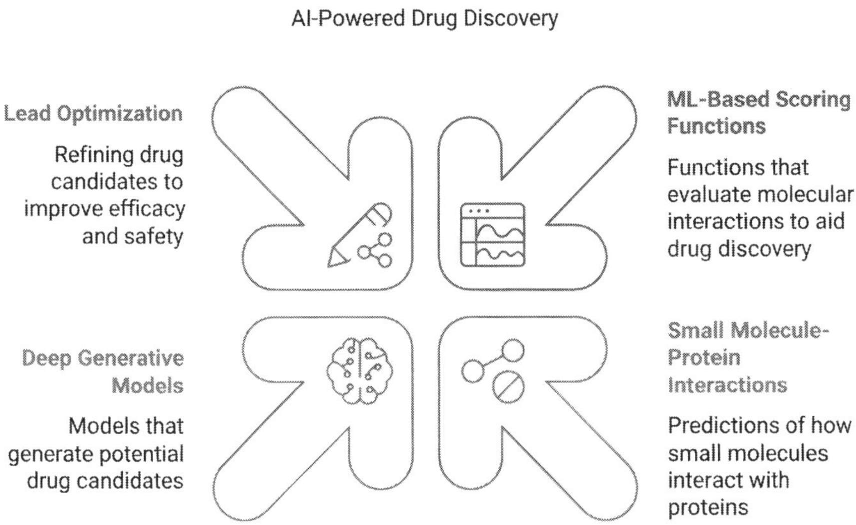

Figure 4.2 Harnessing AI for Next-Generation Drug Discovery

generative capabilities. AI models extract basic molecular patterns from existing bioactive compounds to create novel molecules which have high potential to connect with particular targets [25].

AI also facilitates hit identification and lead optimization by refining molecular structures to improve their binding affinity and pharmacokinetic properties. Advanced feature selection through PCA and unsupervised clustering analysis enables predictive models to pick drug candidates among vast chemical collections. The implementation of AI-based reinforcement learning strategies leads to successive molecular design updates which results in improved drug substance effectiveness together with enhanced safety characteristics.

By integrating AI into virtual screening workflows, researchers can rapidly identify potential drug candidates, validate target interactions, and optimize lead compounds with unprecedented efficiency [26]. These advancements significantly reduce the reliance on expensive and time-consuming wet-lab experiments, ultimately accelerating the development of novel therapeutics (Figure 4.2).

Integrating Real-World Data for AI Target Discovery

Real-world data (RWD) integration represents a revolutionary method which AI employs during drug target discovery. Patient records alongside wearable device outputs and Internet of Things (IoT) health metrics make up RWD which functions as an extensive and dynamic information source to find new drug targets. AI-driven models leverage these diverse datasets to uncover hidden patterns, predict disease progression, and improve drug repurposing strategies. The ability of AI to process vast amounts of real-world evidence (RWE) enhances the precision and efficiency of drug discovery, making treatments more personalized and effective [27].

AI-Driven Analysis of Electronic Health Records (EHRs)

The EHR system maintains structured and unstructured clinical data through patient records, including diagnoses and prescriptions and both diagnostic imaging results and laboratory findings. NLP and ML algorithms powered by AI eliminate meaningful information from these databases to determine new drug-disease connections. By analyzing large-scale EHR data, AI models can detect trends in drug response, uncover adverse drug reactions, and discover new therapeutic applications for existing drugs [28].

Furthermore, predictive modeling of drug response in patient populations has emerged as a critical application of AI in target discovery. AI models use patient genomic data alongside environmental conditions and lifestyle information and medical history to forecast how a person might react to medications. The method supports researchers to create specific treatments and helps with clinical study participant selection and decreases unwanted side effects during therapy while achieving improved outcomes. DL models, such as transformer-based architectures, are increasingly being used to enhance the precision of predictive analytics, thereby facilitating more accurate target identification and validation.

Wearable and IoT Data for Target Discovery

Real-time patient data from IoT-enabled devices and wearable technologies teamed with AI allow researchers to discover targets through unprecedented opportunities. Smartwatches along with biosensors and mobile health applications produce frequent high-frequency measurements of patient physiological and behavioral responses which include heart rate variability and sleep patterns and glucose levels and physical activity information [29]. AI models analyze this longitudinal patient data to detect early biomarkers of disease, predict disease progression, and identify novel drug targets (Figure 4.3).

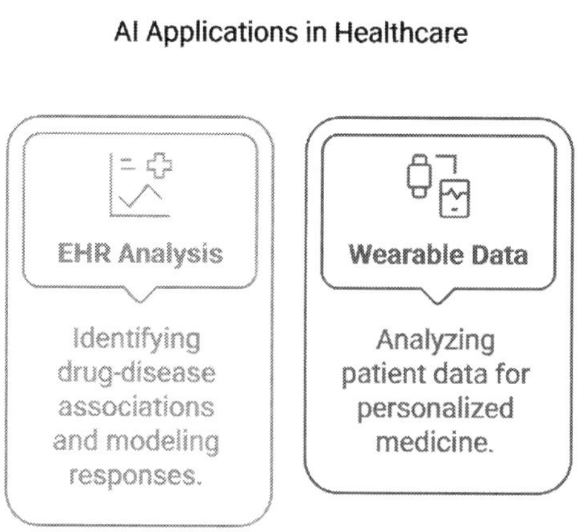

Figure 4.3 AI Applications in Healthcare

Personalized medicine approaches are significantly enhanced through AI-driven biomarker identification from wearable and IoT data. ML algorithms process multi-modal data streams to distinguish normal physiological variations from disease-specific patterns. Modern healthcare benefits from the availability of timely intervention methods that lead to superior clinical trial patient categorization and improved customized therapeutic medical treatments. The implementation of federated learning provides secure methodology for AI-based analysis of dispersed healthcare data without jeopardizing privacy levels and delivers benefits from analyzing extensive aggregated datasets to find new drug targets [30].

By integrating RWD from EHRs, wearables, and IoT devices, AI has the potential to revolutionize drug target identification. The progress in these areas enables researchers to depart from generic treatment discovery methods toward precise therapy methods which results in superior treatment quality and better health outcomes.

Challenges and Ethical Considerations in AI-Driven Drug Target Discovery

The application of AI in drug target identification offers unprecedented advancements in efficiency, accuracy, and scalability. As AI technologies advance it becomes necessary to resolve major obstacles alongside ethical problems for appropriate and ethical deployment. The successful implementation of AI-driven techniques to process genomic data depends heavily on resolving problems involving data bias as well as model interpretability alongside regulatory compliance and ethical standards and fair practices [31].

Data Bias and Model Interpretability

One of the fundamental challenges in AI-driven drug target discovery is data bias. Bias in training datasets, whether due to demographic imbalances, inconsistent data sources, or incomplete biological information, can lead to misleading predictions and incorrect drug target prioritization. The use of AI models trained largely with data from particular populations creates limits in their application across different patient demographics which produces discrepancies in how the drugs affect and affect safety for patients. The resolution of this challenge depends on strenuous data cleaning procedures and inclusive dataset construction methods combined with repetitive assessment of model outputs for discrimination signals [32].

Model interpretability is another critical challenge. Many AI models, particularly DL-based approaches, operate as "black boxes," making it difficult for researchers and regulators to understand how a particular decision was reached. Explainable AI (XAI) techniques, such as Shapley Additive Explanations (SHAP), Local Interpretable Model-agnostic Explanations (LIME), and attention mechanisms in neural networks, are being developed to enhance transparency. The methods provide scientists with tools to better understand AI generated information along with methods to verify predicted drug targets and establish trust in computational pipelines. The enhanceability of AI models makes them reveal not just predictions but it provides detailed scientific explanations about disease processes and drug compound relations [33].

Regulatory and Ethical Considerations

AI-driven drug target discovery must adhere to stringent regulatory guidelines to ensure safety, efficacy, and compliance with international standards. The U.S. Food and Drug Administration (FDA) and EMA have started creating evaluation processes for AI-based pharmaceutical development methods. An organization must fulfill these regulations by recording data origins while testing AI models experimentally and clinically before their insights match confirmed medical knowledge. The lack of standardized regulatory frameworks for AI-driven drug discovery remains a challenge, necessitating close collaboration between AI researchers, pharmaceutical companies, and regulatory bodies to define best practices and approval pathways [34].

In genomic data analysis, ethical concerns are particularly pronounced. AI models analyzing genomic data must ensure patient privacy, informed consent, and compliance with data protection laws, such as the General Data Protection Regulation (GDPR) and the Health Insurance Portability and Accountability Act (HIPAA). Strict ethical oversight becomes imperative to prevent the wrong usage of AI in genomic research which includes illegitimate genetic profiling practices as well as discriminatory activities related to genetic risk elements. Scientists today debate who has rightful control of genomic data because this property might belong to patients while others argue that institutions or developers should own it. Implementing secure data-sharing frameworks, such as federated learning and blockchain-based genomic data management, can help address these concerns while ensuring AI models benefit from diverse and comprehensive datasets [35].

By addressing these challenges and ethical considerations, AI-driven drug target discovery can progress in a responsible and equitable manner. Drug discovery and precision medicine can fully revolutionize through AI because their success depends on maintaining transparency and regulatory compliance and ensuring fairness and ethical integrity.

Future Trends in AI-Based Target Identification

The field of AI-driven drug target identification is rapidly evolving, with emerging technologies pushing the boundaries of computational drug discovery. Target identification will be revolutionized by three innovations known as quantum computing and federated learning and generative AI models which build upon AI integration with advanced computational methods. New advancements in drug discovery technology create more specific and efficient pharmaceutic processes that scale up operations while tackling complexities related to data protection and complex computations and novel target forecasting [36].

Quantum Computing for Molecular Simulations

One of the most promising advancements in AI-based target identification is the integration of quantum computing for molecular simulations. The computational power needed for classical molecular docking along with molecular dynamics simulations proves too extensive to accurately model complex biomolecular interactions. Through quantum mechanics, quantum computing presents a fundamental change that enables precise and fast molecular interaction simulation.

AI-quantum hybrid models are being developed to enhance target identification, particularly for highly intricate biological systems, such as protein-ligand binding interactions and conformational changes in disease-related proteins. These models leverage quantum ML algorithms to solve complex optimization problems that classical AI models struggle with. For example, quantum-enhanced AI approaches can refine drug-binding affinity predictions, optimize molecular conformations, and simulate reaction pathways at a quantum scale. The advancement of quantum hardware makes the combination of quantum computing with AI-based drug target discovery more feasible which advances precision medicine opportunities [37].

Federated Learning for Multi-Center AI Collaboration

A major challenge in AI-driven drug discovery is data sharing between institutions due to privacy concerns and regulatory constraints. Federated learning represents an emerging AI technique that empowers different research facilities along with pharmaceutical organizations and healthcare entities to collectively build AI frameworks through data collaboration without disclosing protected information directly. The distributed training system of federated learning enables AI models to operate on decentralized data collections through security measures that protect sensitive information.

This privacy-preserving AI approach is particularly beneficial in multi-center collaborations for drug target identification, where data from diverse patient populations and biomedical research centers can be leveraged to improve model generalizability. A combination of AI-based drug discovery operations with federated learning enables scientists to build highly performing models which find targets linked to diseases across different datasets within HIPAA-GDPR compliance parameters. The method promotes worldwide drug discovery partnerships through secure patient information management and barriers reduction for dataset accessibility [38].

AI-Enabled De Novo Target Discovery

Generative AI models are transforming the landscape of target identification by predicting novel disease-associated targets with minimal human intervention. Current drug discovery processes employ known biological information together with experimental testing methods to detect targets but the process requires prolonged efforts and stays within established biological pathways. Using AI-powered ways for discovering new drug targets utilizes DL algorithms to generate de novo targets from unexplored biological processes by using both GANs and transformer-based architectures [39].

For example, AI models trained on multi-omics data can generate hypotheses about previously uncharacterized proteins, regulatory elements, or metabolic pathways that may be linked to disease progression. ML models process huge biological data collections of genetic and molecular datasets to search for new therapeutic targets. The AI-assisted process of hypothesis generation delivers exceptional value for difficulties which traditional methods cannot solve due to their rarity and complexity [40].

As AI continues to evolve, integrating quantum computing, federated learning, and generative AI into drug target discovery will reshape the future of precision medicine. The developed tools will boost drug development performance while revealing hidden disease mechanisms, which enables the creation of more precise and beneficial therapeutic approaches.

References

1. Khanna, I. (2012). Drug discovery in pharmaceutical industry: Productivity challenges and trends. *Drug Discovery Today*, *17*, 1088–1102.
2. Strohbehn, G. W., Kacew, A. J., Goldstein, D. A., Feldman, R. C., & Ratain, M. J. (2021). Combination therapy patents: A new front in evergreening. *Nature Biotechnology*, *39*, 1504–1510.
3. Aminabee, S. K., Prabhakar, M. C., Prasad, R. G. S. V., & Lakshmana Rao, A. (2011). Screening the pharmacological activity of cerium oxide nanoparticles in-vitro. *Biomedical and Pharmacology Journal*, *4*(2), 287–289.
4. Chen, W., Liu, X., Zhang, S., & Chen, S. (2023). Artificial intelligence for drug discovery: Resources, methods, and applications. *Molecular Therapy - Nucleic Acids*, *31*, 691–702.
5. Kneller, R. (2010). The importance of new companies for drug discovery: Origins of a decade of new drugs. *Nature Reviews Drug Discovery*, *9*, 867–882.
6. Aminabee, S. K., Lakshmana Rao, A., Sowmya, K., Nymisha, D., Kusuma Naga Lakshmi, K., Manikanta, K. V. N. S., & Praveen Kumar, P. (2019). Evaluation of analgesic activity of *Ficus palmata*. *Iranian Journal of Pharmaceutical Sciences*, *15*(3), 47–60.
7. Brown, D. G., Wobst, H. J., Kapoor, A., Kenna, L. A., & Southall, N. (2022). Clinical development times for innovative drugs. *Nature Reviews Drug Discovery*, *21*, 793–794.
8. Ecker, D. J., Aiello, C. D., Arron, J. R., Bennett, C. F., Bernard, A., Breakefield, X. O., Broderick, T. J., Callier, S. L., Canton, B., & Chen, J. S., et al. (2024). Opportunities and challenges for innovative and equitable healthcare. *Nature Reviews Drug Discovery*, *23*, 321–322.
9. Deng, J., Yang, Z., Ojima, I., Samaras, D., & Wang, F. (2022). Artificial intelligence in drug discovery: Applications and techniques. *Briefings in Bioinformatics*, *23*, bbab430.
10. Chakraborty, C., Bhattacharya, M., & Lee, S. S. (2023). Artificial intelligence enabled ChatGPT and large language models in drug target discovery, drug discovery, and development. *Molecular Therapy - Nucleic Acids*, *33*, 866–868.
11. Aminabee, S. K., Lakshmana Rao, A., & Chinna Eswaraiah, M. (2020). In-vivo antioxidant activity of different fractions of *Indigofera barberi* against paracetamol-induced toxicity in rats. *Turkish Journal of Pharmaceutical Sciences*, *17*(2), 136–140.

12. Paul, D., Sanap, G., Shenoy, S., Kalyane, D., Kalia, K., & Tekade, R. K. (2021). Artificial intelligence in drug discovery and development. *Drug Discovery Today*, *26*, 80–93.
13. Ramesh, A. N., Kambhampati, C., Monson, J. R. T., & Drew, P. J. (2004). Artificial intelligence in medicine. *Annals of the Royal College of Surgeons of England*, *86*, 334–338.
14. Prasanth, D. S. N. B. K., Aminabee, S. K., Lakshmana Rao, A., Teja, N., Bhargavi, K., Monika, C., Pujitha, B., Sandhya, T., Lalitha, A., & Siva Prasad, P. (2020). Anthelmintic activity of *Mansoa alliacea* against *Pheretima posthuma*: In-vitro and in-silico approach. *Thai Journal of Pharmaceutical Sciences*, *4*(3), 186–196.
15. Vamathevan, J., Clark, D., Czodrowski, P., Dunham, I., Ferran, E., Lee, G., Li, B., Madabhushi, A., Shah, P., Spitzer, M., & Zhao, S. (2019). Applications of machine learning in drug discovery and development. *Nature Reviews Drug Discovery*, *18*, 463–477.
16. Sadybekov, A. V., & Katritch, V. (2023). Computational approaches streamlining drug discovery. *Nature*, *616*, 673–685.
17. Askr, H., Elgeldawi, E., Aboul Ella, H., Elshaier, Y. A. M. M., Gomaa, M. M., & Hassanien, A. E. (2023). Deep learning in drug discovery: An integrative review and future challenges. *Artificial Intelligence Review*, *56*, 5975–6037.
18. Prasanth, D. S. N. B. K., Aminabee, S. K., Lakshmana Rao, A., Guntupalli, C., Reddy, A. R., Kulandaivelu, U., Rao, S. N. K., & Rajeshwari, P. (2021). Inhibitory effects of *Mansoa alliacea* in Freund's adjuvant arthritis on inflammatory markers and its confirmation by in-silico strategy. *Thai Journal of Pharmaceutical Sciences*, *45*(6), 532–544.
19. Zdrazil, B., Felix, E., Hunter, F., Manners, E. J., Blackshaw, J., Corbett, S., de Veij, M., Ioannidis, H., Lopez, D. M., & Mosquera, J. F., et al. (2024). The ChEMBL database in 2023: A drug discovery platform spanning multiple bioactivity data types and time periods. *Nucleic Acids Research*, *52*, D1180–D1192.
20. Chen, J., Swamidass, S. J., Dou, Y., Bruand, J., & Baldi, P. (2005). ChemDB: A public database of small molecules and related chemoinformatics resources. *Bioinformatics*, *21*, 4133–4139.
21. Aminabee, S. K., Santhi Krupa, D., Hanumanth Rao, K., Sirisha, V., Anitha Kumari, V., Nagasen, D., Sujiya, B., & Leelavati, T. S. (2023). Pharmacoeconomic analysis of biologic vs. biosimilar therapies in rheumatoid arthritis. *International Journal of Chemical and Biochemical Sciences*, *24*(4), 395–400.
22. Chen, J. H., Linstead, E., Swamidass, S. J., Wang, D., & Baldi, P. (2007). ChemDB update - full-text search and virtual chemical space. *Bioinformatics*, *23*, 2348–2351.
23. Szklarczyk, D., Gable, A. L., Nastou, K. C., Lyon, D., Kirsch, R., Pyysalo, S., & Bork, P. (2021). The STRING database in 2021: Customizable protein-protein networks, and functional characterization of user-uploaded gene/measurement sets. *Nucleic Acids Research*, *49*(D1), D605–D612.
24. Li, X., Tang, Q., Meng, F., Du, P., & Chen, W. (2022). INPUT: An intelligent network pharmacology platform unique for traditional Chinese medicine. *Computational and Structural Biotechnology Journal*, *20*, 1345–1351.
25. Campillos, M., Kuhn, M., Gavin, A. C., Jensen, L. J., & Bork, P. (2008). Drug target identification using side-effect similarity. *Science*, *321*(5886), 263–266.
26. Mendez, D., Gaulton, A., Bento, A. P., Chambers, J., De Veij, M., Félix, E., …, & Hersey, A. (2019). ChEMBL: Towards direct deposition of bioassay data. *Nucleic Acids Research*, *47*(D1), D930–D940.
27. Leelavati, T. S., Madhavi, S., Kamal, G., Raju, P. V. M., Susmitha, K., Vinod, M., & Aminabee, S. K. (2023). Revolutionizing healthcare delivery: Telemedicine's influence on access and patient satisfaction. *International Journal of Chemical and Biochemical Sciences*, *24*(5), 106–115.
28. Kim, S., Chen, J., Cheng, T., Gindulyte, A., He, J., He, S., & Bolton, E. E. (2021). PubChem in 2021: New data content and improved web interfaces. *Nucleic Acids Research*, *49*(D1), D1388–D1395.

29. Sorokina, M., Merseburger, P., Rajan, K., Yirik, M. A., & Steinbeck, C. (2021). COCONUT online: Collection of Open Natural Products database. *Journal of Cheminformatics*, *13*(1), 2.
30. Aminabee, S. K., Devi Mallika, K., & Lakshmana Rao, A. (2023). Natural resources in management and treatment of diseases: A review. *Pharma Times*, *55*(11), 7–10.
31. Wishart, D. S., Feunang, Y. D., Guo, A. C., Lo, E. J., Marcu, A., Grant, J. R., …, & Wilson, M. (2018). DrugBank 5.0: A major update to the DrugBank database for 2018. *Nucleic Acids Research*, *46*(D1), D1074–D1082.
32. Vatansever, S., Schlessinger, A., Wacker, D., Kaniskan, H. Ü., Jin, J., Zhou, M. M., & Zhang, B. (2021). Artificial intelligence and machine learning-aided drug discovery in central nervous system diseases: State-of-the-art and future directions. *Medicinal Research Reviews*, *41*(3), 1427–1473.
33. Aminabee, S. K., & Lakshmana Rao, A. (2024). Computational identification of selected bioactive compounds from *Cedrus deodara* as inhibitors against SARS-CoV-2 main protease: A pharmacoinformatics study. *Indian Drugs*, *61*(2), 78–91.
34. Talevi, A., Morales, J. F., Hather, G., Podichetty, J. T., Kim, S., Bloomingdale, P. C., …, & Wurpel, J. N. D. (2020). Machine learning in drug discovery and development part 1: A primer. *CPT: Pharmacometrics & Systems Pharmacology*, *9*(3), 129–142.
35. Celebi, M. E., & Aydin, K. (2016). *Unsupervised learning algorithms*. Springer International Publishing.
36. Lo, Y. C., Senese, S., France, B., Gholkar, A. A., Damoiseaux, R., & Torres, J. Z. (2017). Computational cell cycle profiling of cancer cells for prioritizing FDA-approved drugs with repurposing potential. *Scientific Reports*, *7*, 11508.
37. Lo, Y. C., Rensi, S. E., Torng, W., & Altman, R. B. (2018). Machine learning in chemoinformatics and drug discovery. *Drug Discovery Today*, *23*(8), 1538–1546.
38. Alloghani, M., Al-Jumeily, D., Mustafina, J., Hussain, A., & Aljaaf, A. J. (2020). A systematic review on supervised and unsupervised machine learning algorithms for data science. In M. W. Berry, A. Mohamed & B. W. Yap (Eds.), *Supervised and unsupervised learning for data science* (pp. 3–21). Springer International Publishing.
39. Xiao, Y. D., Clauset, A., Harris, R., Bayram, E., Santago, P. II, & Schmitt, J. D. (2005). Supervised self-organizing maps in drug discovery. 1. Robust behavior with overdetermined data sets. *Journal of Chemical Information and Modeling*, *45*(6), 1749–1758.
40. Xu, Z., Wang, S., Zhu, F., & Huang, J.. (2017). Seq2seq fingerprint: An unsupervised deep molecular embedding for drug discovery. In *Proceedings of the 8th ACM International Conference on Bioinformatics, Computational Biology, and Health Informatics* (pp. 285–294). ACM.

5 AI in Drug Design and Optimization

Introduction to AI-Driven Drug Design

The landscape of drug discovery underwent significant transformation through Artificial Intelligence (AI) because this technology improved the efficiency of hit identification along with lead optimization and de novo drug design. Multi-year extensive research together with substantial funding requirements and great expense characterize conventional pharmaceutical innovation because it needs multiple clinical trial stages to convert compounds into marketable products. AI-driven approaches, powered by machine learning (ML) and deep learning (DL) algorithms, have addressed these challenges by leveraging large-scale chemical and biological datasets to enhance drug design, improve efficiency, and reduce attrition rates in drug development pipelines [1].

One main benefit of AI drug design incorporates its ability to assess extensive molecular databases and generate accurate predictions of drug candidates that outperform standard computational analysis methods. The training of ML and DL models with chemical structures and bioactivity profiles and pharmacokinetic properties allows them to discover suitable molecular scaffolds and make them more effective and selective while maintaining safety. AI-based drug design integrates both structure-based and ligand-based methodologies, ensuring that novel compounds possess the desired physicochemical and pharmacological properties.

De novo drug design, one of the most revolutionary aspects of AI in pharmacology, enables the generation of novel molecules with optimal properties using generative models. Techniques, such as Generative Adversarial Networks (GANs) and Variational Autoencoders (VAEs), facilitate the creation of entirely new chemical entities that fit specific target profiles. AI-based generative systems use their capability to examine large numbers of possible chemical compounds to create improved drug-like molecules for experimental synthesis and validation [2]. The automation conducted by AI leads to substantial decreases in the duration needed to conduct initial stages of drug research.

The AI technique of reinforcement learning (RL) uses agents that improve molecular structures through feedback analysis of their predicted therapeutic

DOI: 10.4324/9781003616177-5

effect and drug absorption properties. RL-based algorithms enable simultaneous improvement of several drug characteristics, including potency together with solubility and metabolic stability and toxicity assessment. This multi-objective optimization framework ensures that AI-designed drugs strike a balance between therapeutic efficacy and pharmacokinetic suitability, increasing their chances of clinical success.

AI allows scientists to connect different forms of biological datasets, including genomics and transcriptomics and proteomics to determine disease processes while seeking new drug targets. Target-based drug discovery benefits from this systems biology methodology through its ability to reveal complete information about molecular relations and disease progression. AI also plays a crucial role in polypharmacology, where it identifies compounds that can interact with multiple biological targets, leading to more effective and safer therapeutics [3].

Drug design utilizing AI is encountering difficulties due to data bias as well as challenges around achieving understanding of AI models and compliance restrictions. Numerous AI algorithms base their operations on historical datasets, yet these files might include bias which leads to less-than-optimal prediction results. Additionally, explainability in AI models remains a crucial aspect, as black-box models lack transparency in decision-making processes. Regulatory agencies, such as the FDA and EMA, are working toward establishing guidelines for AI-driven drug development to ensure safety, efficacy, and ethical considerations.

Drug discovery research will benefit from upcoming AI advancements through its combination with quantum computing and federated learning technology. The combination of quantum computing with molecular simulation and federated learning system enables powerful complex interaction optimization along with distributed data management that safeguards patient privacy in collaborative medical research [4]. AI is undeniably revolutionizing the pharmaceutical industry, paving the way for a more efficient, cost-effective, and precise approach to drug design and optimization.

AI-Enabled De Novo Drug Design

De novo drug design refers to the creation of novel molecular structures from scratch, guided by specific pharmacokinetic and pharmacodynamic requirements. The process has been transformed by AI through its ability to create new molecules using advanced computational approaches of GANs and VAEs and RL.

Generative Adversarial Networks (GANs) for Molecular Generation

GANs consist of two neural networks – a generator and a discriminator that compete against each other to create new molecular structures with high synthetic feasibility. The generator creates new chemical compounds and the discriminator validates them using learned chemical knowledge together with drug-friendly properties. As the adversarial process continues its work the molecular generator improves its capabilities to produce varied versatile compounds which are suitable for synthesis [5]. GANs are particularly useful in designing lead compounds with enhanced bioactivity while avoiding undesirable characteristics, such as high toxicity or poor solubility.

Variational Autoencoders (VAEs) for Structural Diversity

VAEs are DL models that learn a compressed representation of chemical structures, allowing them to generate new molecules based on existing patterns and trends in chemical space. The continuous latent space mapping of known drug-like molecules allows VAEs to create compound collections with various structures and optimized PK and PD profiles simultaneously. The use of VAEs extends exploration into uncharted chemical structures past traditional drug libraries, which results in superior possibilities for identifying treatments against complex diseases. Additionally, VAEs can integrate multi-objective optimization techniques to ensure that newly generated molecules meet specific design criteria, such as bioavailability, stability, and target selectivity [6].

Reinforcement Learning (RL) for Optimized Drug Candidates

RL further enhances AI-driven de novo drug design by enabling the iterative optimization of drug candidates based on predefined reward functions. ML based on RL performs active exploration of new chemical compounds and molecular structure refinement through real-time feedback instead of depending on statistical historical data. The RL algorithms grant rewards for molecules that demonstrate excellent target affinity and favorable ADME characteristics while being synthetically accessible. By continuously adjusting molecular structures in response to feedback, RL models can optimize multiple molecular attributes simultaneously, accelerating the lead optimization process (Figure 5.1).

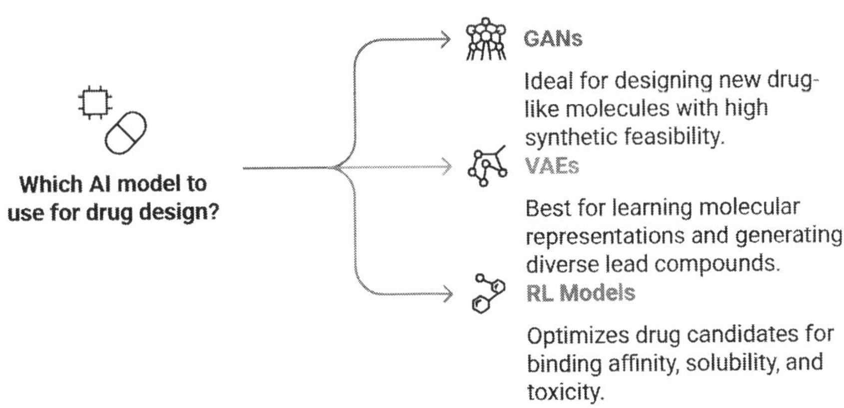

Figure 5.1 AI Model for Drug Design

Advantages of AI in De Novo Drug Design

The integration of AI-driven generative models has revolutionized drug discovery by overcoming several key challenges [7]:

- *Rapid Exploration of Chemical Space:* Traditional drug discovery relied on limited chemical libraries, whereas AI-generated molecules can be designed de novo, offering a broader range of potential drug candidates.
- *Cost and Time Efficiency:* AI-driven models reduce the reliance on costly and time-consuming wet-lab experiments by predicting molecular properties in silico before synthesis.
- *Personalized Drug Development*: AI-generated molecules can be tailored based on patient-specific genetic and biochemical profiles, enabling precision medicine approaches.

AI-Driven Structure-Based Drug Design (SBDD)

Modern drug discovery heavily relies on Structure-Based Drug Design (SBDD) as a vital approach which AI-driven methods improve drug candidate screening and refinement processes and their efficiency. AI uses DL models in combination with graph-based representations along with protein structure prediction breakthroughs to accomplish exact drug-target interaction modeling. The new innovations help speed up the discovery of hit compounds while minimizing expenses spent during traditional discovery workflows [8].

AI-Powered Molecular Docking

Molecular docking is a fundamental technique in SBDD that predicts the binding interactions between small molecules (ligands) and target proteins. AI-powered molecular docking improves upon traditional docking methods by integrating DL-based scoring functions, which evaluate the binding affinity and stability of ligand-protein complexes with higher accuracy. AI-driven docking models analyze extensive biochemical datasets through predictive analyses to obtain greater effectiveness in the prediction of binding interactions when compared to classical docking approaches that use empirical scoring functions. Such models enhance docking precision through their ability to handle molecular adaptability while considering solvent interactions and protein-ligand movement patterns to efficiently select top-quality drug molecules [9].

Graph Neural Networks (GNNs) for Binding Affinity Prediction

GNNs have revolutionized molecular property prediction by capturing intricate molecular topological features. In the context of SBDD, GNNs model the structural relationships between atoms and bonds within a molecule, allowing for more precise binding affinity predictions. The dynamic learning process of

GNNs generates molecular representations through which they can accurately determine drug-binding interactions with proteins. GNNs enable discovery of new ligands with superior pharmacokinetic properties through analysis of extensive biochemical information libraries. GNNS improve virtual screening by selecting compounds based on their ability to bind efficiently and their ADMET quality features [10].

AlphaFold and Protein Structure Prediction

The advent of AlphaFold, an AI-powered protein structure prediction model, has transformed SBDD by providing near-atomic resolution models of protein structures. Understanding a protein's three-dimensional (3D) conformation is essential for designing drugs that precisely fit into its active site. AlphaFold alongside other DL-based protein folding models enhances protein structure modeling accuracy which allows scientists to predict protein structures that were formerly unresolvable. Such an advancement improves ligand-binding predictions because researchers can develop more rational drug design programs. AI-driven protein structure prediction also facilitates the discovery of allosteric binding sites, which can be targeted for modulating protein function in a disease-specific manner (Figure 5.2).

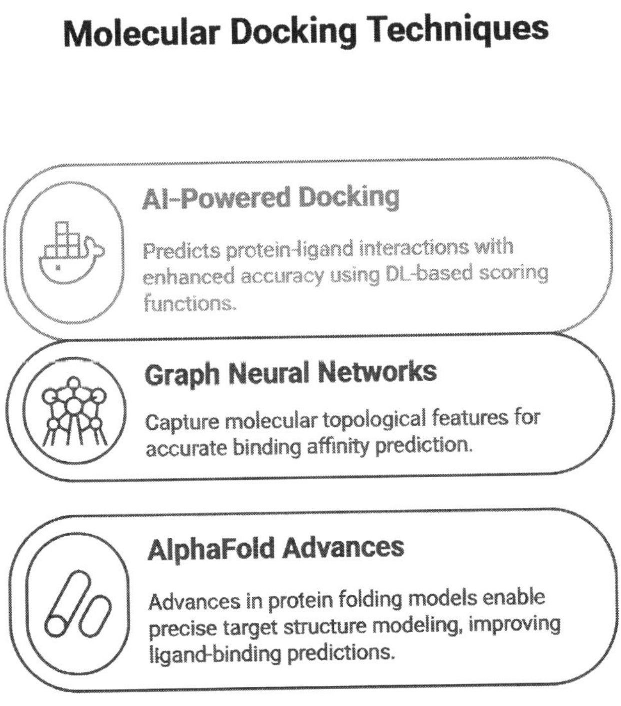

Figure 5.2 AI-Driven Structure-Based Drug Design

Advantages of AI-Driven SBDD

AI-powered SBDD offers several advantages over conventional drug design approaches:

- *Enhanced Binding Affinity Predictions:* AI models learn from vast experimental datasets, improving the accuracy of docking simulations and reducing false positives.
- *Accelerated Virtual Screening*: AI-driven molecular docking enables the rapid screening of millions of compounds, significantly expediting the identification of potential drug candidates.
- *Improved Target Flexibility Consideration*: AI models incorporate protein dynamics and conformational changes, addressing limitations of rigid docking techniques.
- *Discovery of Novel Drug-Binding Sites:* AI-driven structural analysis reveals new allosteric and cryptic sites for innovative drug design strategies (Table 5.1).

Table 5.1 AI-Driven Structure-Based Drug Design Approaches

AI Technique	*Application in SBDD*	*Advantages*	*Challenges*
AI-Powered Molecular Docking	Predicts protein-ligand interactions with enhanced accuracy using deep learning-based scoring functions.	• Higher accuracy in binding affinity predictions • Improved virtual screening outcomes	• False positives in docking predictions • Requires extensive labeled datasets
Graph Neural Networks (GNNs)	Captures molecular topology to predict binding affinity and drug-target interactions.	• Learns from complex molecular structures • Improves virtual screening efficiency	• Requires large-scale biochemical datasets • Computationally intensive
AlphaFold & Protein Structure Prediction	Provides high-accuracy 3D models of protein structures, improving target-based drug discovery.	• Enhances drug-target interaction modeling • Identifies novel allosteric sites	• Does not always account for ligand-induced conformational changes
Hybrid AI-Physics-Based Models	Combines AI and physics-based simulations for precise molecular interactions.	• Reduces computational cost compared to traditional simulations • Improves accuracy in predicting real-world interactions	• Limited availability of experimental validation data
Reinforcement Learning for SBDD	Optimizes molecular docking and ligand binding through iterative learning.	• Enables adaptive learning for drug optimization • Improves hit-to-lead transition efficiency	• Requires fine-tuning to avoid bias in learning algorithms

AI for Multi-Objective Drug Optimization

AI-driven approaches have transformed multi-objective drug optimization by addressing key challenges in balancing efficacy, safety, and pharmacokinetics. Drugs developed through traditional discovery techniques restrict their efforts to enhance one characteristic (potency), thus creating medical safety or bioavailability challenges. Parameters optimization through AI models delivers simultaneous assessments, which enhances lead optimization frameworks and speeds up the conversion of initial drug candidates to disease-fighting drugs [11].

Multi-Parameter Optimization (MPO)

Multi-Parameter Optimization (MPO) is a computational approach that integrates multiple drug-related properties, including potency, selectivity, solubility, metabolic stability, and toxicity, into a unified optimization framework. AI-based MPO models assess a vast chemical space, predicting the likelihood of a compound meeting all required criteria for clinical success. AI-powered MPO operates through predictive modeling together with RL, which conducts dynamic improvements of molecular structures without needing traditional trial-and-error processes. The models cut down the number of late stage drug development failures through their ability to pick compounds that maintain acceptable pharmacokinetic and pharmacodynamic ratios [12].

Bayesian Optimization

Bayesian optimization is a probabilistic method used to refine molecular designs efficiently by balancing exploration (searching new chemical spaces) and exploitation (refining known promising candidates). The system implements two components to estimate the objective function (drug efficacy) by creating surrogate models which direct the selection of next promising compounds for testing through acquisition functions. Through uncertainty estimation, Bayesian optimization improves lead optimization, so AI systems can choose molecules which show maximum potential for success. This method reduces the number of experimental iterations required to identify optimal drug candidates, making the drug discovery process more resource-efficient [13].

Pareto Front-Based AI Models

Pareto front-based AI models are used to identify compounds that achieve the best possible trade-offs among multiple drug attributes, such as potency, bioavailability, and toxicity. These models generate a Pareto front consisting of multiple non-dominated solutions because no single parameter achievement could happen without trade-offs with other parameters. Drugs under development are optimized using evolutionary algorithms in conjunction with deep RL and graph-based neural networks which locate them on the Pareto front [14]. This approach enables researchers to make informed decisions by selecting compounds with the best balance of desirable properties, increasing the likelihood of clinical success (Table 5.2).

Table 5.2 AI for Multi-Objective Drug Optimization

AI Technique	*Description*	*Key Benefits*
Multi-Parameter Optimization (MPO)	AI-driven approach to balance multiple drug properties, such as efficacy, safety, and pharmacokinetics.	Ensures drug candidates meet multiple criteria simultaneously, improving success rates.
Bayesian Optimization	Uses probabilistic models to guide the selection of molecules based on uncertainty estimation.	Enhances lead optimization by efficiently exploring chemical space, reducing experimental costs.
Pareto Front-Based AI Models	Identifies compounds that provide the best trade-offs between potency, bioavailability, and toxicity.	Enables rational decision-making by selecting candidates with optimal balance across multiple objectives.

AI in Polypharmacology and Drug Repurposing

AI has significantly advanced the field of polypharmacology, which focuses on the interaction of drugs with multiple targets, and drug repurposing, which aims to find new therapeutic uses for existing drugs. Traditional drug discovery practices adopt a "one drug, one target" approach yet AI-driven research allows proper identification of multi-target drugs that treat complex conditions, such as cancer alongside neurodegenerative disorders and infectious diseases. The integration of vast biological datasets together with off-target effect prediction and drug-disease relationship discovery makes AI an enabler of polypharmacological research [15].

AI-Powered Target Affinity Prediction

AI-driven target affinity prediction models leverage DL and ML algorithms to analyze drug-target interactions across multiple biological pathways. The models integrate molecular docking simulations alongside chemical structure embeddings together with omics data integration to discover drugs which bind to many targets. AI's ability to predict drug affinities proves essential for managing diseases, including Alzheimer's and cancer, since multiple-target therapy provides better therapeutic benefit due to complex pathophysiology. By improving drug-target interaction predictions, AI helps optimize combination therapies and reduce adverse effects associated with single-target treatments [16].

Network Pharmacology Models

AI-driven network pharmacology utilizes computational methods to analyze large-scale biological networks, mapping relationships between drugs, targets, and diseases. By uniting data obtained from both genomics and proteomics and transcriptomics and metabolomics, these models seek new therapeutic applications for drugs already established. The integration of AI into drug-disease association network construction enables researchers to identify promising repurposing candidates for high translation effectiveness. AI-based network pharmacology proves valuable for personalized treatments because it can establish customized drug interactions that combine individual genetic along with molecular specifics [17].

Transfer Learning for Drug Repurposing

Transfer learning, a subfield of DL, enhances drug repurposing by allowing AI models trained in one therapeutic domain to be adapted to new disease contexts. The application of pretrained AI models enables the use of datasets for learning drug molecule properties to make efficacy and safety predictions about different diseases. Drug repurposing processes become faster through the implementation of this approach because it decreases the requirement for large-scale de novo drug screening tests [18]. AI-based transfer learning has successfully identified novel applications for drugs like metformin, originally developed for diabetes but now being explored for cancer treatment (Figure 5.3).

AI in ADMET Prediction and Toxicity Assessment

The integration of AI in Absorption, Distribution, Metabolism, Excretion, and Toxicity (ADMET) prediction has significantly enhanced drug discovery by improving the accuracy and efficiency of pharmacokinetic and toxicological assessments. Drug-likeness predictions alongside safety profiles become feasible through large biological chemical and clinical datasets processed by AI models which decreases the occurrence of late stage drug failures.

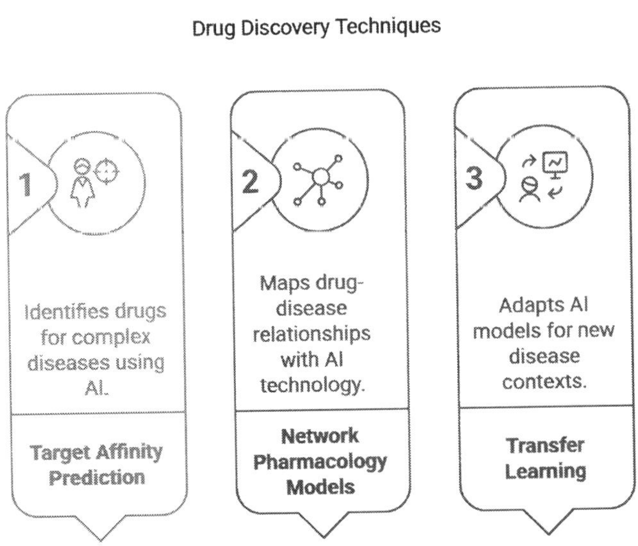

Figure 5.3 AI in Polypharmacology and Drug Repurposing

AI-Based ADMET Models for Drug-Likeness Prediction

The evaluation of drug candidates with key pharmacokinetic properties through AI-driven ADMET models occurs with ML, DL together with graph-based algorithms. Through predictive analysis AI tools display the manner by which drugs are taken up by the body and how they distribute to tissues while revealing their breakdown by liver enzymes and approve both kidney and liver exits and their toxic potentials. Quantitative Structure-Activity Relationship (QSAR) models, convolutional neural networks (CNNs), and recurrent neural networks (RNNs) analyze molecular descriptors to assess drug-likeness [19]. By filtering out compounds with poor ADMET properties early, AI reduces development costs and enhances the selection of viable drug candidates.

AI-Driven Virtual Screening for Toxicity Assessment

AI has transformed toxicology screening by predicting hepatotoxicity, cardiotoxicity, nephrotoxicity, and neurotoxicity before in vivo testing. DL models, trained on databases such as Tox21, PubChem, and OpenTG-GATEs, analyze structural and biological data to identify compounds with adverse effects. The evaluation of drug-target interactions together with metabolic stability and off-target effects through in silico toxicology models determined by AI helps prevent clinical trial failures. DeepTox together with ToxCast utilize neural networks for predicting toxicity results through molecular fingerprints analysis [20].

AI Models for Hepatotoxicity and Cardiotoxicity Prediction

Hepatotoxicity (liver toxicity) remains a leading cause of drug withdrawals. AI models assess the likelihood of a drug causing liver damage by analyzing its metabolic pathways, interactions with hepatic enzymes, and potential to form toxic metabolites. AI models analyze drug interactions with human Ether-à-go-go-Related Gene channels to monitor heart toxicity and predict cardiotoxicity through such channels that regulate cardiac functions. AI sensors that predict hERG liability assist medical staff to find compounds with dangerous heart behavior therefore enhancing drug testing security.

AI for Metabolism and Drug-Drug Interaction (DDI) Predictions

Metabolism plays a crucial role in drug efficacy and safety. AI-based models predict cytochrome P450 (CYP) enzyme interactions, which determine how a drug is metabolized and cleared from the body. The combination of cheminformatics data with metabolomics and transcriptomics data through AI enhances forecasts related to metabolic stability together with drug-drug interactions and pharmacokinetic properties [21]. ML models use their capabilities to transform molecular structures for better metabolic features, which raises the probability of drug approval.

Explainable AI (XAI) for Regulatory Toxicology

Regulatory agencies, such as the Food and Drug Administration (FDA) and European Medicines Agency (EMA), require transparency in AI-driven ADMET predictions. XAI techniques offer explanations about model decision processes to fulfill regulatory requirements. SHAP alongside LIME along with attention-based neural networks provide researchers a means to determine which molecular components affect toxicity prediction outputs. This transparency improves trust in AI models for clinical applications and regulatory approvals.

Future Directions in AI-Driven ADMET Predictions

The future of AI in ADMET modeling lies in multi-modal learning, federated AI, and quantum-enhanced toxicity predictions. Predictive accuracy in personalized medicine will improve through AI systems that use actual clinical data together with patient-derived organoids as well as wearable biosensor information. The combination of AI-quantum hybrid systems works to optimize toxicity prediction by modeling atomic-scale molecular interactions. The continuing advancements will enhance both the reliability and the efficiency of AI systems applied to pharmacokinetics as well as drug safety assessment tasks [22].

AI and Quantum Computing in Drug Design

Drug discovery benefits today from AI collaboration with quantum computing through efficient molecular simulations alongside optimized drug-target interactions. Traditional computational methods often struggle with complex molecular modeling due to high-dimensional data and computational limitations. However, quantum computing, when combined with AI, offers a powerful solution by efficiently solving molecular interaction problems at an atomic level.

Quantum Machine Learning (QML) in Drug Discovery

Quantum Machine Learning (QML) enhances molecular simulations by combining quantum algorithms with AI-driven models. The method delivers fast analyses of high-dimensional chemical venues in addition to allowing researchers to optimize molecular structures that create better predictions of drug-related properties, including solubility permeability and toxicity. QML implements a process that cuts down the time needed to evaluate drug candidates as part of early stage drug development process acceleration [23].

Hybrid AI-Quantum Models for Molecular Interactions

Hybrid AI-quantum models are revolutionizing the understanding of drug-target interactions. Traditional molecular docking techniques base their operations on classical computing systems yet experience difficulties in predicting dynamic movements of molecules. The binding affinity prediction capabilities of

AI-quantum hybrid models are enhanced through quantum simulations which deliver detailed explanations regarding drug-biological target interactions. The models perform dual functions of structuring molecules to achieve better performance while developing less harmful outcomes.

Quantum Chemistry and AI for Lead Optimization

Quantum chemistry plays a crucial role in drug discovery by predicting the stability and electronic properties of molecules. Quantum models powered by AI process quantum mechanical evaluations to identify reactive molecular behaviors and measure binding energy levels for selecting lead compounds. Quantum-enhanced DL when applied by researchers allows them to identify better drug candidates featuring desirable pharmacokinetic alongside pharmacodynamic characteristics, thus raising clinical trial success rates [24].

Future Perspectives and Challenges in AI-Driven Drug Design

The future of AI in drug discovery holds immense potential, with emerging technologies addressing critical challenges in pharmaceutical research. Medical drug progress becomes faster through AI technology but operational barriers emerge from data protection matters together with moral concerns and supervisory requirements. The combination of federated learning with advances in AI fairness and better regulatory compliance defines the evolving principles of drug development conducted with AI assistance.

Federated Learning in Drug Discovery

Federated learning is a decentralized AI approach that enables multiple research institutions, pharmaceutical companies, and hospitals to collaboratively train AI models without directly sharing sensitive patient data. This technique optimizes drug-target interaction predictions in discovery operations through secure information protection. The distributed AI system of federated learning avoids noncompliance with strong data security rules, such as GDPR and HIPAA. Such an approach benefits drug development by uniting diverse healthcare insights from around the world, thus eliminating bias and strengthening the accuracy of AI predictions [25].

Ethical Considerations and AI Bias

AI models used in drug discovery rely on vast datasets that may carry inherent biases related to demographics, ethnicity, or disease prevalence. The continued existence of outdated biological assumptions will produce an uneven drug development process which provides superior treatment options to one group at the expense of others. Fair AI prediction results stem from bias reduction when organizations adopt audit methodology and explainable AI approaches together with multiple training data sources. Additionally, ethical concerns related to AI-generated molecules, including intellectual property rights and biosecurity risks, must be addressed to foster responsible AI-driven drug design.

Regulatory Challenges in AI Drug Discovery

Despite AI's transformative impact on pharmaceutical research, regulatory agencies, such as the FDA and EMA, have yet to fully establish guidelines for AI-designed drugs. Some AI models operate as black boxes, thus creating barriers for validating molecular candidates developed by AI before clinical trials. Health authorities need to develop updated guidelines which bring AI-based pharmaceutical research into alignment with security protocols and performance benchmarks as well as moral standards [26]. AI-assisted regulatory submissions combined with real-world AI validation studies will serve as critical tools for making progress in the acceptance of AI by regulatory authorities.

The integration of AI into pharmaceutical research hinges on resolving present challenges for the future development of AI applications in drug discovery. Letting AI address data privacy together with ethical considerations and regulatory compliance standards will transform the development process for new therapeutic treatments, thus enabling superior patient results across worldwide healthcare systems.

References

1. Ramesh, A. (2004). Artificial intelligence in medicine. *Annals of the Royal College of Surgeons of England*, *86*(5), 334–338.
2. Aminabee, S. K., Prabhakar, M. C., Prasad, R. G. S. V., & Lakshmana Rao, A. (2011). Screening the pharmacological activity of cerium oxide nanoparticles in-vitro. *Biomedical and Pharmacology Journal*, *4*(2), 287–289.
3. Miles, J., & Walker, A. (2006). The potential application of artificial intelligence in transport. *IEE Proceedings – Intelligent Transport Systems*, *153*(2), 183–198.
4. Yang, Y., & Siau, K. (2018). A qualitative research on marketing and sales in the artificial intelligence age. In MWAIS 2018 Proceedings.
5. Aminabee, S. K., Lakshmana Rao, A., Sowmya, K., Nymisha, D., Kusuma Naga Lakshmi, K., Manikanta, K. V. N. S., & Praveen Kumar, P. (2019). Evaluation of analgesic activity of *Ficus palmata*. *Iranian Journal of Pharmaceutical Sciences*, *15*(3), 47–60.
6. Smith, R. G., & Farquhar, A. (2000). The road ahead for knowledge management: An AI perspective. *AI Magazine*, *21*(4), 17.
7. Lamberti, M. J. (2019). A study on the application and use of artificial intelligence to support drug development. *Clinical Therapeutics*, *41*(8), 1414–1426.
8. Aminabee, S. K., Lakshmana Rao, A., & Chinna Eswaraiah, M. (2020). In-vivo antioxidant activity of different fractions of *Indigofera barberi* against paracetamol-induced toxicity in rats. *Turkish Journal of Pharmaceutical Sciences*, *17*(2), 136–140.
9. Beneke, F., & Mackenrodt, M.-O. (2019). Artificial intelligence and collusion. *International Review of Intellectual Property and Competition Law*, *50*(2), 109–134.
10. Steels, L., & Brooks, R. (2018). *The artificial life route to artificial intelligence: Building embodied, situated agents*. Routledge.
11. Prasanth, D. S. N. B. K., Aminabee, S. K., Lakshmana Rao, A., Teja, N., Bhargavi, K., Monika, C., Pujitha, B., Sandhya, T., Lalitha, A., & Siva Prasad, P. (2020). Anthelmintic activity of *Mansoa alliacea* against *Pheretima posthuma*: In-vitro and in-silico approach. *Thai Journal of Pharmaceutical Sciences*, *4*(3), 186–196.

12. Vyas, M. (2018). Artificial intelligence: The beginning of a new era in pharmacy profession. *Asian Journal of Pharmaceutics, 12*(2), 72–76.
13. Duch, W. (2007). Artificial intelligence approaches for rational drug design and discovery. *Current Pharmaceutical Design, 13*(14), 1497–1508.
14. Prasanth, D. S. N. B. K., Aminabee, S. K., Lakshmana Rao, A., Guntupalli, C., Reddy, A. R., Kulandaivelu, U., Rao, S. N. K., & Rajeshwari, P. (2021). Inhibitory effects of *Mansoa alliacea* in Freund's adjuvant arthritis on inflammatory markers and its confirmation by in-silico strategy. *Thai Journal of Pharmaceutical Sciences, 45*(6), 532–544.
15. Sellwood, M. A. (2018). Artificial intelligence in drug discovery. *Future Medicinal Chemistry, 10*(17), 2025–2028.
16. Zhu, H. (2020). Big data and artificial intelligence modeling for drug discovery. *Annual Review of Pharmacology and Toxicology, 60*, 573–589.
17. Aminabee, S. K., Santhi Krupa, D., Hanumanth Rao, K., Sirisha, V., Anitha Kumari, V., Nagasen, D., Sujiya, B., & Leelavati, T. S. (2023). Pharmacoeconomic analysis of biologic vs. biosimilar therapies in rheumatoid arthritis. *International Journal of Chemical and Biochemical Sciences, 24*(4), 395–400.
18. Ciallella, H. L., & Zhu, H. (2019). Advancing computational toxicology in the big data era by artificial intelligence: Data-driven and mechanism-driven modeling for chemical toxicity. *Chemical Research in Toxicology, 32*(3), 536–547.
19. Chan, H. S. (2019). Advancing drug discovery via artificial intelligence. *Trends in Pharmacological Sciences, 40*(8), 592–604.
20. Leelavati, T. S., Madhavi, S., Kamal, G., Raju, P. V. M., Susmitha, K., Vinod, M., & Aminabee, S. K. (2023). Revolutionizing healthcare delivery: Telemedicine's influence on access and patient satisfaction. *International Journal of Chemical and Biochemical Sciences, 24*(5), 106–115.
21. Firth, N. C. (2015). MOARF, an integrated workflow for multiobjective optimization: Implementation, synthesis, and biological evaluation. *Journal of Chemical Information and Modeling, 55*(6), 1169–1180.
22. Ravi Shankar, K., Aminabee, S. K., Ramana, G., Chenchu Lakshmi, K. N. V., & Indusree, G. (2024). Formulation and evaluation of propranolol hydrochloride floating tablets by 32 factorial design. *International Journal of Drug Delivery Technology, 14*(4), 2060–2067.
23. Zhang, L. (2017). From machine learning to deep learning: Progress in machine intelligence for rational drug discovery. *Drug Discovery Today, 22*(11), 1680–1685.
24. Aminabee, S. K., Devi Mallika, K., & Lakshmana Rao, A. (2023). Natural resources in management and treatment of diseases: A review. *Pharma Times, 55*(11), 7–10.
25. King, R. D. (1995). Comparison of artificial intelligence methods for modeling pharmaceutical QSARs. *Applied Artificial Intelligence, 9*(3), 213–233.
26. Aminabee, S. K., & Lakshmana Rao, A. (2024). Computational identification of selected bioactive compounds from *Cedrus deodara* as inhibitors against SARS-CoV-2 main protease: A pharmacoinformatics study. *Indian Drugs, 61*(2), 78–91.

6 Preclinical and Clinical Development Using AI

Introduction

The integration of artificial intelligence (AI) in drug development has transformed traditional methodologies by enhancing the speed, accuracy, and efficiency of preclinical and clinical research. Previous drug discovery processes lasted very long while costing extensive money while delivering low success rates. Computer-assisted innovations transform these procedures by letting data-based decisions and predictive modeling and automation. The development cycle of pharmaceutical products using AI technologies, including machine learning (ML), deep learning (DL), and natural language processing (NLP), now determines optimal medication identification along with evaluation and optimized drug modification procedures as well as security and effectiveness assessments [1].

In preclinical development, AI accelerates the identification of novel drug candidates through multi-omics data analysis, structure-based drug design, and in silico toxicity prediction. AI-driven molecular simulations, combined with quantum computing, allow researchers to explore vast chemical spaces and predict drug-target interactions with unprecedented accuracy. The AI-powered microphysiological systems (MPS) known as organ-on-a-chip technologies create human-based simulations that reduce animal testing and improve the preclinical data translation to human outcomes. Through federated learning, organizations can create secure systems that let multiple sites collaborate on data sharing and protect individual privacy elements, thus encouraging inclusive preclinical drug development at a worldwide level.

In clinical research, AI is streamlining clinical trial design, patient recruitment, and outcome prediction. Traditional clinical trials face challenges, such as high costs, lengthy timelines, and difficulties in patient stratification. AI-based patient selection through the combination of EHRs and real-world data will direct trials to enroll the optimal patients, which leads to higher success rates. DCTs enabled through AI-empowered remote monitoring of patients with wearable devices create greater inclusion for participants while enhancing their commitment to studies and minimizing delivery problems [2]. Synthetic control arms built from AI-produced patient information instead of placebo groups help enhance trial efficiency and handle ethical concerns.

DOI: 10.4324/9781003616177-6

Beyond clinical trials, AI plays a pivotal role in post-market surveillance through advanced pharmacovigilance systems. AI-driven algorithms analyze real-world evidence, social media, and electronic health records to detect adverse drug reactions (ADRs) early, allowing for prompt regulatory interventions. Regulatory document preparation using AI integration together with automated literature review services simplifies the approval procedures by maintaining adherence to international guidelines, such as those of the FDA and EMA. The integration of AI with quantum computing is set to further revolutionize drug development by enhancing molecular simulations, optimizing personalized medicine approaches, and refining dose-response predictions.

Despite its transformative potential, AI-driven drug development faces significant challenges. Widespread adoption of AI faces significant challenges because of the problems that stem from unintelligible models along with biased AI predictions and regulatory authorization barriers. The need for robust AI governance systems becomes fundamental because ethical factors around data privacy and algorithmic clarity as well as biased decision processes create issues involving privacy [3]. Ongoing progress regarding explainable AI (XAI) and federated learning methods together with AI models that adhere to regulations will solve these problems.

The future of AI in preclinical and clinical development lies in the seamless integration of AI with cutting-edge technologies, such as quantum computing, real-world evidence analytics, and precision medicine. The pharmaceutical sector can decrease drug creation expenses and shorten development periods while boosting treatment success rates along with medicine safety through AI automation along with predictive methods.

AI in Preclinical Drug Development

AI-Powered Target Identification

The process of identifying drug targets is a critical step in drug discovery, as it involves pinpointing molecular entities, such as proteins, genes, or pathways, that play a crucial role in disease pathology. The current methodology for target identification includes three sequential steps that demand lengthy experimentation and expensive asset usage. The combination of AI with multi-omics data analysis and advanced computational models and ML predictive analytics tools boosts the accuracy and efficiency of this process. AI-powered target identification utilizes DL, graph neural networks (GNNs), and single-cell sequencing to uncover novel therapeutic targets with high precision [4].

Deep Learning-Based Multi-Omics Analysis

DL algorithms are revolutionizing target identification by integrating and analyzing large-scale multi-omics data, including genomics, transcriptomics, proteomics, and metabolomics. By analyzing biological data patterns correctly these models generate a complete understanding of disease mechanisms. AI systems use convolutional neural networks (CNNs) alongside recurrent neural networks (RNNs) to assess genetic mutations with gene expression profiles together with protein interactions for developing forecasts about new druggable targets. For instance, DL models trained on cancer genomic data can identify oncogenes and tumor suppressors that drive tumor progression, leading to the discovery of highly specific drug targets [5]. AI's multi-omics analysis capabilities help researchers obtain disease phenotype-disease genetic correlation associations to identify intervention targets that traditional analysis methods cannot detect.

Graph Neural Networks (GNNs) for Gene-Disease Association Prediction

GNNs have emerged as a powerful AI-driven tool for understanding gene-disease relationships. The GNN architecture represents biological interactions through electronic graphs that connect functional elements which consist of genes and proteins and diseases through corresponding edges. Large biological network training for GNNs results in predictions of new genetic-disease associations, which leads to the discovery of unexplored drug objectives. These models are particularly useful in rare and complex diseases, where traditional approaches struggle to identify genetic contributors. GNNs have been successfully applied to reconstruct disease-associated gene networks, predict pathogenic mutations, and infer mechanistic links between genetic variations and disease progression [6]. A learning system based on GNNs derives its reliable capability to detect targets due to its ability to process diverse biological datasets.

AI-Driven Single-Cell RNA Sequencing (scRNA-seq) for Precision Target Discovery

Single-cell RNA sequencing (scRNA-seq) provides a high-resolution view of gene expression at the individual cell level, offering unprecedented insights into cellular heterogeneity in diseases, such as cancer, neurodegenerative disorders, and autoimmune diseases. The integration of AI analysis in scRNA-seq leads to improved drug target recognition through its capability to analyze similar profiles of gene expression patterns and its ability to identify uncommon cell groups as well as anticipate cell developmental pathways. Traditional bulk RNA sequencing averages gene expression across many cells, potentially masking crucial disease-driving genes that are active only in specific subpopulations. AI models examine large volumes of single-cell transcriptomic datasets to determine both pathway dysregulation and disease-regulating cellular factors. This precise methodology benefits immunotherapy research because it enables AI systems to detect both tumor-specific antigens and immune checkpoint regulators for developing patient-specific treatment plans [7].

AI-Enhanced Epigenomic Mapping for Drug Resistance Mechanisms

Epigenetic modifications, such as DNA methylation and histone modifications, play a significant role in gene regulation and drug resistance. AI-based epigenomic

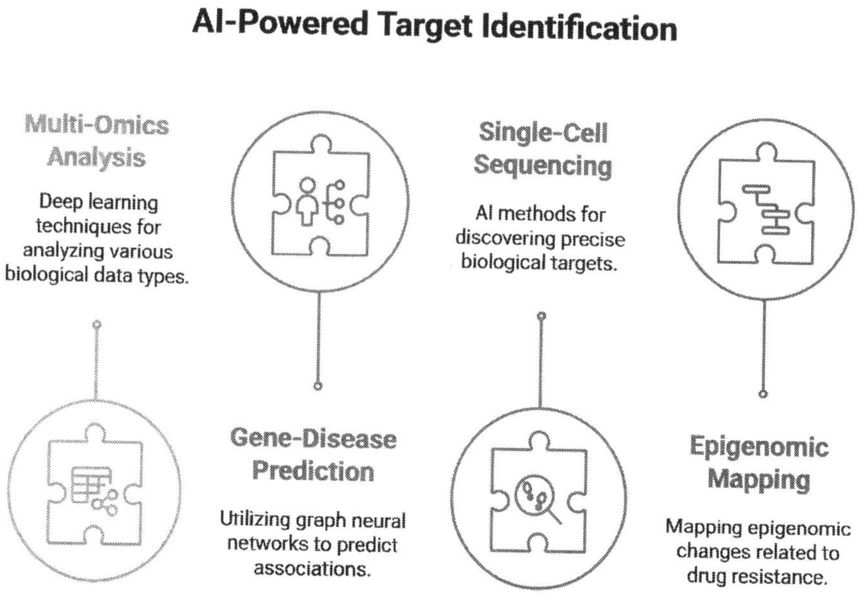

Figure 6.1 AI-Powered Target Identification

analysis allows scientists to track epigenetic transformations between disease states which helps them determine influential regulatory components that result in drug resistance. Computer programs trained with epigenomic data predict both enhancer-promoter connections and chromatin accessibility features together with histone modifications linked to persistent cancers. AI analysis of epigenetics provides essential knowledge about cancer cell response to drug treatment which helps scientists develop resistance-combating treatment approaches [8]. By integrating AI with chromatin immunoprecipitation sequencing (ChIP-seq) and ATAC-seq data, researchers can identify novel epigenetic drug targets, leading to the development of combination therapies that reprogram resistant cancer cells (Figure 6.1).

AI-Driven Lead Optimization and Drug Design

Lead optimization is a critical phase in drug discovery, where promising lead compounds undergo refinement to enhance their pharmacokinetic, pharmacodynamic, and safety profiles. The drug development method formerly used sequential medicinal chemistry transformations which were steered by experimental data and understanding of structure-activity relationships (SAR). This approach requires numerous resources and takes extensive time while also failing to recognize the complete molecular complex structures effectively. Drugs become more effective and show reduced toxicity with fewer off-target effects because AI optimizes lead structures during the design phase [9]. AI-driven approaches, such as generative models, self-supervised learning, quantum-enhanced AI, and deep reinforcement learning (DRL), are transforming the way drugs are designed and optimized.

Generative AI for De Novo Drug Molecule Generation

Generative AI, powered by DL architectures, such as variational autoencoders (VAEs) and generative adversarial networks (GANs), has revolutionized the design of novel drug molecules from scratch. The drug discovery methods using traditional chemical libraries screening become obsolete since generative AI builds new molecular designs which adhere to preset pharmaceutical requirements. The models absorb knowledge from extensive drug-like chemical data to produce newly designed compounds that fulfill essential characteristics, including binding capacity and dissolution capability and biological availability. By employing reinforcement learning techniques, generative AI can refine molecule generation based on real-time feedback from molecular simulations and experimental data [10]. This approach drastically reduces the time required for hit identification and enables the rapid discovery of structurally diverse and highly potent lead compounds.

Self-Supervised Learning for Predictive ADMET Modeling

One of the key challenges in lead optimization is ensuring that candidate molecules possess favorable pharmacokinetic properties while minimizing toxicity risks. AI-driven self-supervised learning models have emerged as powerful tools for predictive Absorption, Distribution, Metabolism, Excretion, and Toxicity (ADMET) profiling. The models utilize large chemical structure and biological activity datasets to project new compound effects in biological environments. AI algorithms that work self-supervised overcome limitations of conventional rule-based ADMET systems because they discover intricate molecular patterns between structures and biological outcomes even when operating without large labeled datasets [11]. Advanced neural networks, such as graph convolutional networks (GCNs) and transformer-based architectures, enhance the accuracy of ADMET predictions, enabling researchers to prioritize drug candidates with optimal safety and efficacy profiles before preclinical testing.

Quantum-Enhanced AI for Molecular Docking and Ligand Optimization

Molecular docking plays a crucial role in drug design by predicting the binding affinity between a drug candidate and its target protein. Classic docking systems execute computationally pricey processes while failing to address molecular interaction's dynamic attributes. The integration of quantum computing with AI has introduced a paradigm shift in molecular docking and ligand optimization. Using quantum mechanics-based simulations quantum-enhanced AI models performs molecular interaction predictions at an elevated precision level. The solution of complicated Schrodinger equations turns out to be quicker through these models, which opens up bigger space for chemical exploration for finding ideal lead compound binding arrangements [12]. Research teams attain better binding specificity together with reduced off-target effects through drug stability improvement by implementing quantum-enhanced AI systems with DL capabilities. This approach has significant implications for developing drugs targeting challenging proteins, such as intrinsically disordered proteins and membrane-bound receptors.

Deep Reinforcement Learning (DRL) for Structure-Based Drug Design

DRL has emerged as a cutting-edge AI technique for structure-based drug design, where the molecular structure of the target protein is used to guide drug optimization. The learning process of DRL algorithms takes place through molecular interaction along with reward-based assessments of drug-likeness and bindings affinity as well as pharmacokinetic properties rather than using standard supervised learning datasets. AI agents operate inside these models to automatically search through chemical compounds and learn through successive testing phases, which enhances molecular structure quality. DRL-driven drug design has been particularly effective in optimizing lead compounds for challenging drug targets, such as protein-protein interactions (PPIs) and allosteric sites [13]. By adapting itself continuously, DRL achieves timely optimization of drug molecules to fulfill multiple design requirements, such as potency together with selectivity and metabolic stability (Figure 6.2).

AI in Preclinical Testing and Safety Assessment

Preclinical testing is a critical phase in drug development, aimed at evaluating a compound's efficacy, pharmacokinetics, and safety before it progresses to clinical trials. Drugs and their toxic effects traditionally get evaluated through the combination of cell cultures studied in test tubes and animal studies conducted in live subjects. These testing approaches face various drawbacks, such as ethical challenges and differences between species and their expense when used in research. The integration of AI in preclinical testing and safety assessment has revolutionized this phase by enhancing predictive accuracy, reducing reliance on animal testing, and

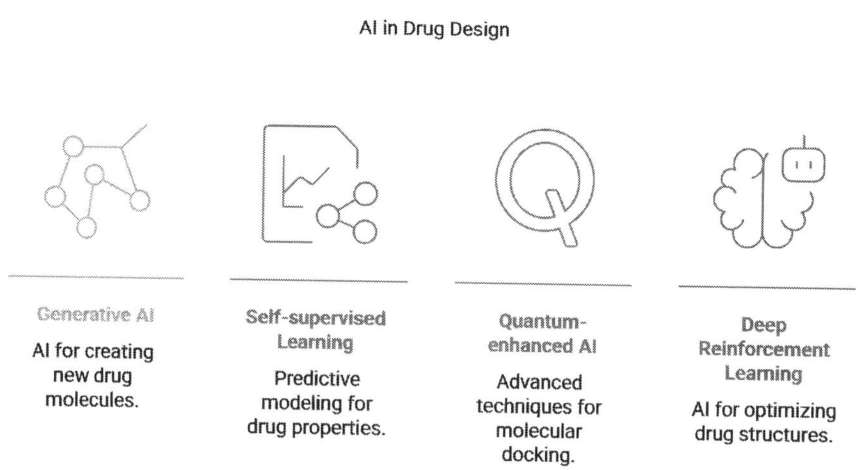

Figure 6.2 AI-Driven Lead Optimization and Drug Design

expediting drug evaluation. The drug assessment process faces a transformation through the implementation of AI-powered MPS together with digital twin models with omics-based toxicology and federated learning [14].

AI-Powered Microphysiological Systems (MPS) and Organ-on-a-Chip Models

MPS, also known as organ-on-a-chip models, are advanced in vitro platforms that mimic the physiological and functional properties of human organs. The microfluidic technology enables researchers to build three-dimensional (3D) human tissue environments which present more precise drug evaluation than traditional cell cultures. AI elevates MPS safety assessments by adding current data evaluation paired with predictive models along with ML structures that optimize drug assessment outcomes. AI-driven image processing tools analyze cellular morphology, biochemical signals, and physiological responses within these systems, providing detailed insights into drug-induced toxicity, metabolism, and organ-specific effects [15]. AI-powered MPS enable researchers to both decrease animal experimentation needs and produce preclinical research outcomes of superior clinical value.

Digital Twin Models for Simulating Preclinical Drug Response

Digital twin technology is emerging as a groundbreaking AI application in preclinical drug testing. Digital twins represent virtual copies of biological systems that emerge from patient-unique and statistical population information. These AI models create simulated simulations which reproduce drug responses as well as disease advancement along with toxicity profiles at an individualized level. In preclinical studies, digital twins enable the simulation of drug interactions with various physiological systems, allowing researchers to predict adverse effects, optimize dosing regimens, and refine candidate selection before conducting laboratory experiments. Additions of fresh experimental observations help digital twins develop progressively improved predictive models [16]. This technological advancement shortens preclinical assessment duration and minimizes expenditure to improve both drug safety prediction outcomes.

AI-Driven Omics-Based Toxicology and Histopathological Analysis

Omics-based approaches, including genomics, transcriptomics, proteomics, and metabolomics, have revolutionized toxicology by providing molecular-level insights into drug-induced effects. Computational models based on AI process intricate omics information to detect toxicity patterns and discover biochemical warning signs of medication safety issues and determine how drugs affect different individuals. The analysis of large multi-omics datasets by ML algorithms creates molecular-toxicity associations which allow medical staff to recognize potential safety threats beforehand. Additionally, AI-powered histopathological analysis automates the assessment of tissue samples from preclinical studies. DL models trained on large datasets of histopathological images can detect subtle morphological changes indicative of drug-induced toxicity with high accuracy [17].

By implementing AI-driven techniques the accuracy of toxicity evaluations improves along with the elimination of manual labors that used to consume excessive time.

Federated Learning for Multi-Institutional Preclinical Collaborations

Federated learning is an advanced AI approach that allows multiple institutions to collaborate on preclinical research without sharing raw data. This training method supports distributed AI model development within different research institutions along with pharmaceutical operations and academic frameworks through protected information safeguards. The drug development process for preclinical studies benefits from federated learning by uniting multiple organizations to share different data collections, including drug responses and toxicity parameters and disease modeling results. By leveraging collective intelligence, AI models trained through federated learning improve their predictive capabilities and generalizability across different biological systems [18]. The joint effort between institutions helps to strengthen preclinical results while speeding up drug safety certifications and supporting evidence-based choices during drug development (Table 6.1).

Table 6.1 AI in Preclinical Drug Development

Category	*AI Technologies and Approaches*	*Applications*
AI-Powered Target Identification	Deep learning-based multi-omics analysis	Integrates genomics, transcriptomics, and proteomics to identify drug targets
	Graph neural networks (GNNs)	Predicts gene-disease associations for target selection
	AI-driven single-cell RNA sequencing (scRNA-seq)	Identifies disease-specific biomarkers and drug targets
	AI-enhanced epigenomic mapping	Detects drug resistance mechanisms through epigenetic changes
AI-Driven Lead Optimization and Drug Design	Generative AI	Designs novel drug molecules for lead identification
	Self-supervised learning for ADMET modeling	Predicts drug absorption, metabolism, and toxicity for optimization
	Quantum-enhanced AI	Enhances molecular docking and ligand optimization
	Deep reinforcement learning (DRL)	Facilitates structure-based drug design for improved efficacy
AI in Preclinical Testing and Safety Assessment	AI-powered microphysiological systems (MPS)	Uses organ-on-a-chip models for in vitro drug testing
	Digital twin models	Simulates preclinical drug responses for toxicity assessment
	AI-driven omics-based toxicology	Analyzes transcriptomics and proteomics for safety profiling
	Federated learning	Enables data sharing across institutions while preserving privacy

AI in Clinical Development

AI for Clinical Trial Optimization

Clinical trials are the cornerstone of drug development, determining the safety and efficacy of new treatments before regulatory approval. The standard clinical trial methods require extended time and heavy expenses because they experience high failure rates because of insufficient patient enrollment and variable datasets and complex regulatory requirements. The implementation of AI in clinical trials brought important improvements to patient selection procedures and boosted both trial efficiency and protected trial data at its sources. AI-powered methodologies, such as synthetic control arms, decentralized clinical trials (DCTs), multi-omics patient stratification, and blockchain-integrated AI, are driving a new era of smarter, faster, and more reliable clinical research [19].

Synthetic Control Arms (SCAs) Using Generative Adversarial Networks (GANs)

One of the major challenges in clinical trials is the recruitment of control groups, particularly in rare diseases or life-threatening conditions where a placebo arm may be unethical. Through AI, the synthetic control arms system creates imitated control groups from historic patient information instead of relying on actual patient enrollment. GANs function as an AI sub-category to generate realistic synthetic patient data through pattern recognition of available clinical datasets. These AI-generated control arms allow for precise comparisons between treatment and control groups while reducing patient recruitment burdens and ethical concerns. SCAs accelerate clinical trials by minimizing delays caused by control arm recruitment, thereby expediting drug approval timelines [20].

AI-Powered Decentralized Clinical Trials (DCTs) with Remote Monitoring

Traditional clinical trials often require patients to visit centralized study sites, posing logistical challenges, such as travel burdens, recruitment inefficiencies, and high dropout rates. AI-based DCTs tackle these issues through digital platforms paired with mobile health applications with biosensors that let participants enroll from remote locations. AI controls remote monitoring systems which gather ongoing healthcare information from patients to aid drug evaluation without needing in-person clinical assessments. NLP algorithms analyze patient-reported outcomes, while ML models detect adverse events early, ensuring timely interventions. AI-driven DCTs integrated by pharmaceutical companies produce better patient retention and trial diversity together with faster data collection which makes trials more precise for patients and operationally efficient [21].

Multi-Omics AI for Adaptive Patient Stratification

Patient heterogeneity often leads to variability in drug responses, making it challenging to design successful clinical trials. The use of AI to run multi-omics analysis of genomics and proteomics and transcriptomics and metabolomics permits doctors to create patient profiles for individual drug prediction based on biomarkers found in data. Multiple ML programs evaluate large data collections from multiomics sources to build genetic and metabolic and molecular patient categories for precise clinical trial applications. This AI-driven patient stratification enhances trial success rates by selecting individuals who are most likely to benefit from a given therapy while minimizing variability in treatment outcomes. AI-powered adaptive trials examine patient data systematically to update trial criteria as well as enhance medication dose schedules and enhance trial impact [22].

Blockchain-Integrated AI for Clinical Data Security

Clinical trials generate vast amounts of sensitive patient data, necessitating robust security measures to ensure data integrity, confidentiality, and regulatory compliance. The combination of AI technology with blockchain functions as a tamper-resistant and decentralized system which handles clinical data management. The combination of AI with blockchain technology provides protected database systems which enable instant check-up of trial information while performing automatic proof checks to stop data modifications and misinformation. Smart contracts powered by AI facilitate transparent and automated regulatory reporting, ensuring compliance with global guidelines, such as Good Clinical Practice (GCP) and the General Data Protection Regulation (GDPR). The implementation of AI-driven blockchain technology leads to better data protection through which stakeholders develop trust and creates more efficient regulatory processes and enhances clinical trial outcome reliability [23].

AI in Pharmacovigilance and Post-Market Surveillance

Pharmacovigilance and post-market surveillance are essential components of drug safety monitoring, ensuring that approved medications continue to be effective and safe for public use. Traditional pharmacovigilance practices depend on manual reporting mechanisms together with spontaneous adverse event submissions and retrospective evaluations because these methods require significant time and produce incomplete data subject to nondetectable reporting. Post-market surveillance has seen a revolution through AI-based technologies which provide instantaneous adverse outcome recognition while conducting predictive safety evaluations and delivering proactive risk mitigation. Innovations, such as NLP, IoT-enabled AI monitoring, AI-driven drug repurposing, and predictive safety models, are significantly enhancing the efficiency and accuracy of pharmacovigilance efforts [24].

Natural Language Processing (NLP) for Adverse Event Detection from EHRs and Real-World Data

ADRs remain difficult to detect from the huge amount of unstructured medical data found in EHRs and social media posts and patient forums as one key obstacle in pharmacovigilance. NLP algorithms equipped with AI analyze multiple data types to find substantial information about drug safety. NLP can identify ADR patterns by scanning medical notes, detecting patient-reported symptoms, and analyzing clinical narratives. Advanced NLP models, including transformer-based architectures like BERT and GPT, can process and interpret complex medical terminology, improving the accuracy of adverse event detection. Through NLP-based pharmacovigilance system adoption regulatory agencies together with pharmaceutical companies gain the ability to identify safety warning signs sooner which speeds up risk control initiatives [25].

IoT-Enabled AI for Real-Time Patient Monitoring and Pharmacokinetics

The Internet of Things (IoT), combined with AI, is transforming post-market drug monitoring by enabling real-time patient health tracking. Healthcare devices with built-in biosensors along with intelligent medical technology connect to mobile applications which continuously monitor heart rates as well as blood pressure recordings and glucose measurements and monitor patient medicine usage and physiological patterns. AI algorithms analyze this real-time data to assess individual drug responses, detect early signs of adverse reactions, and predict potential safety concerns before they escalate. AI-enhanced pharmacokinetic modeling uses IoT-enabled real-time data to create personalized drug dosages and optimal therapeutic plans. The utilization of IoT-enabled AI allows pharmacovigilance teams to switch from safety monitoring only to proactive intervention tactics which ensures better patient safety while enhancing medication adherence [26].

AI-Driven Drug Repurposing and Label Expansion

AI is playing a crucial role in post-market drug repurposing by identifying new therapeutic applications for existing drugs. The difference between generative drug repurposing and AI-powered analysis resides in traditional methods depending on serendipitous findings and clinical observations and AI conducting comprehensive analysis of genomic databases and chemical structures from real-world evidence sources [27]. ML models and DL networks identify novel drug disease associations by recognizing patterns in molecular pathways and patient response data. Additionally, AI-guided label expansion helps pharmaceutical companies expand drug indications by analyzing retrospective clinical trial data and real-world treatment outcomes. The use of AI allows researchers to minimize expense and achieve faster treatment releases while serving patients suffering from untreated medical conditions (Figure 6.3).

Predictive AI Models for Long-Term Drug Safety Assessment

Long-term drug safety assessment is crucial for identifying delayed adverse effects, drug-drug interactions, and cumulative toxicity risks. The current spontaneous reporting system used in post-market surveillance takes extensive amounts of time

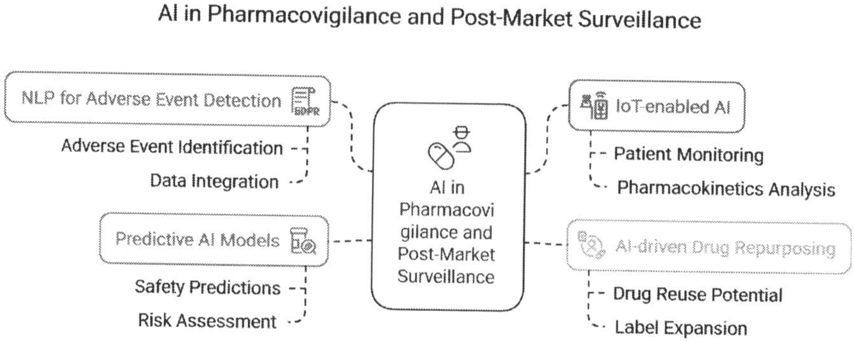

Figure 6.3 AI in Pharmacovigilance and Post-Market Surveillance

to discover both uncommon safety risks and extended-term adverse effects. The combination of predictive modeling fueled by AI solves problems in risk projection by using data from multi-omics analysis and health records with real-world evidence monitoring to find possible drug-related long-term risks. AI models analyze historical adverse event trends, patient demographics, and genetic factors to predict individuals who may be at higher risk for specific side effects. Furthermore, reinforcement learning algorithms continuously refine safety predictions based on emerging clinical data, ensuring that risk assessments remain up to date. The combination of AI predictive pharmacovigilance technology helps regulatory bodies and health providers deploy aimed patient surveillance systems and immediate safety warnings to achieve safer drug management results for population health [28].

AI in Personalized Medicine and Regulatory Compliance

The integration of AI into personalized medicine and regulatory compliance is revolutionizing how drugs are developed, prescribed, and approved. Personalized medicine develops individual treatment plans by incorporating genetic markers with lifestyle considerations together with patients' disease states for precision care through reduced negative side effects. However, achieving true precision medicine requires advanced computational tools to analyze vast amounts of biological and clinical data. AI, particularly in combination with emerging technologies, such as quantum computing and digital twin simulations, is enabling unprecedented levels of customization in treatment regimens. The use of AI for regulatory frameworks enables quick drug approvals and maintains high safety requirements for new medications to reach patients more efficiently [29].

AI-Powered Digital Twin Technology for Individualized Treatment Simulations

One of the most groundbreaking applications of AI in personalized medicine is digital twin technology. The creation of digital twins requires multiscale patient information from omics data combined with actual health records and medical images and vital signs measurements. Research scientists and medical practitioners use AI to operate digital twin simulations for predicting treatment outcomes among specific patients prior to treatment delivery. These simulations can model disease progression, drug metabolism, and potential adverse effects, enabling the selection of the most effective and least harmful therapeutic approach. In oncology, for example, digital twins can predict tumor responses to different chemotherapeutic agents, guiding personalized cancer treatment plans [30]. The advancement of AI model sophistication will boost digital twin technology toward precise patient treatment in therapeutic areas of neurology alongside immunology and cardiology.

Hybrid AI-Quantum Computing for Precision Dose Optimization

Optimizing drug dosage is a complex challenge in personalized medicine, as individuals metabolize and respond to medications differently due to genetic and physiological variations. Traditional dose calculations rely on population-based pharmacokinetics, which may not be optimal for every patient. The combination of AI and ML systems with quantum computing power allows for immediate individual dose optimization through hybrid models. Quantum-enhanced AI can process vast biological datasets simultaneously, analyzing molecular interactions and patient-specific metabolic pathways with unprecedented accuracy. These hybrid models use prediction technologies to help dosage determination for optimal drug effectiveness together with reduced toxicity risk in patient bodies [31]. The approach delivers optimal results when treating medications with limited safe therapeutic space, such as anticoagulants together with immunosuppressants and chemotherapy agents.

Regulatory AI for Streamlined FDA, EMA, and PMDA Approval Processes

The regulatory approval of new drugs is traditionally a lengthy and resource-intensive process, involving extensive clinical trials, safety evaluations, and documentation. The use of AI technology enables efficient regulatory process streamlining that speeds up innovative therapy approvals without leading to safety concerns. The FDA (US) and EMA (Europe) and PMDA (Japan) adopt AI tools to automate data evaluation and detect potential risks and provide faster clinical trial assessment using more efficient processes. AI-driven NLP systems can rapidly scan and summarize regulatory submissions, ensuring compliance with industry standards. Additionally, ML algorithms are being used to predict the success probability of new drug applications, helping pharmaceutical companies refine their strategies before submission. AI continues to make essential contributions to regulatory post-market compliance through its ability to monitor real-world patient data and identify unexpected adverse effects which leads to rapid risk control measures [32].

AI-Enhanced Pharmacogenomics for Personalized Drug Response Prediction

Pharmacogenomics, the study of how genetic variations affect drug response, is a cornerstone of personalized medicine. AI-based pharmacogenomic models use genomic data from patients to forecast drug reactions thereby helping healthcare providers make effective selection decisions about medication choices. AI solves traditional pharmacogenomic challenges by using biological data from various sources, such as proteomics and transcriptomics and genomics. This allows AI to overcome the limitation of incomplete datasets and complex gene-drug interactions. DL models can identify previously unknown genetic markers associated with drug efficacy or adverse reactions, leading to more precise medication recommendations. For instance, AI-powered pharmacogenomic analysis has improved dosing strategies for anticoagulants like warfarin, reduced trial-and-error prescribing in psychiatric medications, and enhanced immunotherapy selection in cancer treatment [33]. The personalized drug therapy approach enabled by AI generates better patient results, which leads to reduced adverse drug effects and higher treatment efficiency rates (Table 6.2).

Table 6.2 AI in Clinical Development

Category	*AI Technologies and Approaches*	*Applications*
AI for Clinical Trial Optimization	Synthetic control arms (SCAs)	Uses GANs to create virtual control groups for reducing trial size
	AI-powered decentralized clinical trials (DCTs)	Enables remote patient monitoring and participation
	Multi-omics AI	Uses genomic and proteomic data for adaptive patient stratification
	Blockchain-integrated AI	Ensures secure and tamper-proof clinical data management
AI in Pharmacovigilance and Post-Market Surveillance	Natural language processing (NLP)	Extracts adverse event reports from EHRs and real-world data
	IoT-enabled AI	Monitors patients in real time for pharmacokinetic analysis
	AI-driven drug repurposing	Identifies new therapeutic indications for existing drugs
	Predictive AI models	Assesses long-term drug safety and adverse event risks
AI in Personalized Medicine and Regulatory Compliance	AI-powered digital twin technology	Simulates individualized treatment responses
	Hybrid AI-quantum computing	Optimizes precision dosing based on patient-specific factors
	Regulatory AI	Streamlines approval processes with FDA, EMA, and PMDA compliance
	AI-enhanced pharmacogenomics	Predicts personalized drug responses based on genetic data

Future Challenges and Perspectives

Explainable AI (XAI) for Regulatory Transparency in Drug Approvals

As AI plays an increasingly vital role in drug discovery and clinical decision-making, regulatory agencies demand greater transparency in AI-driven models. XAI comes forward to meet this requirement through decision-making processes which become transparent to researchers along with clinicians and members of regulatory institutions. DL models which base their operations on traditional neural networks operate as closed systems since they generate accurate results yet fail to demonstrate their reasoning behind decisions. This lack of transparency can hinder regulatory approval and adoption in critical fields, such as medicine [34].

XAI techniques, including attention mechanisms, SHapley Additive Explanations (SHAP) values, and counterfactual reasoning, enable researchers to trace AI-generated predictions back to specific features in the input data. XAI provides drug discovery with understanding of which molecular structure shows high binding affinity to target molecules and explains patient subgroup treatment responses. The FDA together with EMA are developing framework integration programs for XAI which ensures AI-supported drug evaluations proceed through explainable, research-based processes. As AI continues to evolve, XAI will play a pivotal role in ensuring trust, accountability, and regulatory compliance in pharmaceutical innovation.

Bias Mitigation Strategies in AI-Driven Drug Development

AI models draw their functionality from the quality of training data yet biases in education sets can result in drug development delivering biased and unfair results. The introduction of bias to drug discovery via AI originates from three main reasons: imbalanced clinical trial participant demographics and genetic data differences together with uneven disease patient population distribution [35]. When these biases manifest, they produce drugs which underperform or show adverse effects on minority populations while worsening current disparities in healthcare.

To address these concerns, several bias mitigation strategies have been developed. One approach is dataset balancing, ensuring that AI models are trained on diverse and representative patient populations. Through federated learning technique medical institutions maintain patient data privacy by allowing decentralized model learning across various institutions, thus minimizing potential biases caused by single-source data. AI models learn to fight bias while being trained through adversarial debiasing methods during their learning process. Researches can establish fair drug discovery and development through the insertion of algorithms which enhance equitable patient outcomes across various demographics [36].

Quantum-AI Hybrid Models for Next-Generation Drug Discovery

The combination of quantum computing and AI is revolutionizing drug discovery by significantly enhancing molecular modeling, predictive analytics, and optimization processes. The high-dimensionality of chemical space presents challenges for traditional computational methodologies in drug discovery because they need extensive computational power to predict optimal candidates. The capabilities of quantum computing for parallel processing massive dataset quantities now drive revolutionary changes in these processes through advanced computational capabilities.

Quantum-AI hybrid models integrate quantum algorithms with classical AI techniques to optimize molecular docking, predict ligand-binding affinities, and simulate quantum chemical properties with high precision. The execution of quantum simulations becomes more efficient because AI directs researchers toward important molecular structures that both shave down computational expenses and produce more accurate predictions. By using quantum-enhanced AI researchers can speed up drug development through precise models of atomic protein-ligand interactions which brings down lead optimization times [37]. This hybrid approach is particularly valuable for complex drug targets, such as intrinsically disordered proteins or PPIs, which are challenging to analyze using conventional methods. As quantum computing continues to advance, its integration with AI is expected to unlock new frontiers in next-generation drug discovery.

Privacy-Preserving AI Techniques for Clinical Data Sharing

Research and drug development conducted with AI face major privacy issues because patient data should move between institutions while maintaining full compliance with HIPAA and GDPR privacy rules. The current methods of sharing data have problems with exposing valuable patient information which leads to security risks and breaches of confidentiality. Privacy-preserving AI techniques, including federated learning and homomorphic encryption, offer innovative solutions to enable secure and ethical data sharing without compromising privacy.

The AI model training process happens across various healthcare facilities within a federated learning framework without the need for actual patient information transfer. Healthcare institutions work together for model updates on shared AI programs while keeping their data stored at their individual locations. The approach protects data security as it enables institutions to obtain the benefits of numerous large datasets to create more generalized models. Homomorphic encryption gives AI models the power to operate on encrypted clinical data so researchers can study protected medical information through computation without gaining access to it. During the complete analytical process, the data protection stays intact because of this technique [38].

Through privacy-preserving AI approaches pharmaceutical businesses together with healthcare organizations attain improved cooperation during medical research and drug development activities. Through these advancements researchers can improve data security and they gain access to worldwide datasets for developing AI innovations which contribute to better drug outcomes in development and clinical AI implementation speedups.

References

1. Mullard, A. (2021). 2020 FDA drug approvals. *Nature Reviews Drug Discovery*, *20*, 85–90.
2. Brown, D. G., & Wobst, H. J. (2021). A decade of FDA-approved drugs (2010–2019): Trends and future directions. *Journal of Medicinal Chemistry*, *64*, 2312–2338.
3. Fleming, N. (2018). How artificial intelligence is changing drug discovery. *Nature*, *557*, S55–S57.
4. Aminabee, S. K., Prabhakar, M. C., Prasad, R. G. S. V., & Lakshmana Rao, A. (2011). Screening the pharmacological activity of cerium oxide nanoparticles in-vitro. *Biomedical and Pharmacology Journal*, *4*(2), 287–289.
5. Schneider, P., Walters, W. P., Plowright, A. T., Sieroka, N., Listgarten, J., & Goodnow, R. A. Jr. et al. (2020). Rethinking drug design in the artificial intelligence era. *Nature Reviews Drug Discovery*, *19*, 353–364.
6. Schuhmacher, A., Gatto, A., Kuss, M., Gassmann, O., & Hinder, M. (2021). Big techs and startups in pharmaceutical R&D: A 2020 perspective on artificial intelligence. *Drug Discovery Today*, *26*, 2226–2231.
7. Aminabee, S. K., Lakshmana Rao, A., Sowmya, K., Nymisha, D., Kusuma Naga Lakshmi, K., Manikanta, K. V. N. S., & Praveen Kumar, P. (2019). Evaluation of analgesic activity of *Ficus palmata*. *Iranian Journal of Pharmaceutical Sciences*, *15*(3), 47–60.
8. Aoyama, T., Suzuki, Y., & Ichikawa, H. (1990). Neural networks applied to pharmaceutical problems. III. Neural networks applied to quantitative structure-activity relationship (QSAR) analysis. *Journal of Medicinal Chemistry*, *33*, 2583–2590.
9. Klingler, D. E. (1988). Expert systems in the pharmaceutical industry. *Drug Information Journal*, *22*, 249–258.
10. Vignaux, P. A., Minerali, E., Foil, D. H., Puhl, A. C., & Ekins, S. (2020). Machine learning for discovery of GSK3β inhibitors. *ACS Omega*, *5*, 26551–26561.
11. Aminabee, S. K., Lakshmana Rao, A., & Chinna Eswaraiah, M. (2020). In-vivo antioxidant activity of different fractions of *Indigofera barberi* against paracetamol-induced toxicity in rats. *Turkish Journal of Pharmaceutical Sciences*, *17*(2), 136–140.
12. McCloskey, K., Sigel, E. A., Kearnes, S., Xue, L., Tian, X., & Moccia, D. et al. (2020). Machine learning on DNA-encoded libraries: A new paradigm for hit finding. *Journal of Medicinal Chemistry*, *63*, 8857–8866.
13. Stork, C., Chen, Y., Sicho, M., & Kirchmair, J. (2019). Hit Dexter 2.0: Machine-learning models for the prediction of frequent hitters. *Journal of Chemical Information and Modeling*, *59*, 1030–1043.
14. Ain, Q. U., Aleksandrova, A., Roessler, F. D., & Ballester, P. J. (2015). Machine-learning scoring functions to improve structure-based binding affinity prediction and virtual screening. *Wiley Interdisciplinary Reviews: Computational Molecular Science*, *5*, 405–424.
15. Prasanth, D. S. N. B. K., Aminabee, S. K., Lakshmana Rao, A., Teja, N., Bhargavi, K., Monika, C., Pujitha, B., Sandhya, T., Lalitha, A., & Siva Prasad, P. (2020). Anthelmintic activity of *Mansoa alliacea* against *Pheretima posthuma*: In-vitro and in-silico approach. *Thai Journal of Pharmaceutical Sciences*, *4*(3), 186–196.
16. Graff, D. E., Shakhnovich, E. I., & Coley, C. W. (2021). Accelerating high-throughput virtual screening through molecular pool-based active learning. *Chemical Science*, *12*, 7866–7881.
17. Yang, Y., Yao, K., Repasky, M. P., Leswing, K., Abel, R., Shoichet, B. K., & Jerome, S. V. (2021). Efficient exploration of chemical space with docking and deep-learning. *Journal of Chemical Theory and Computation*, *17*, 7106–7119.
18. Paul, S. M., Mytelka, D. S., Dunwiddie, C. T., Persinger, C. C., Munos, B. H., & Lindborg, S. R., et al. (2010). How to improve R&D productivity: The pharmaceutical industry's grand challenge. *Nature Reviews Drug Discovery*, *9*, 203–214.
19. Prasanth, D. S. N. B. K., Aminabee, S. K., Lakshmana Rao, A., Guntupalli, C., Reddy, A. R., Kulandaivelu, U., Rao, S. N. K., & Rajeshwari, P. (2021). Inhibitory effects of

Mansoa alliacea in Freund's adjuvant arthritis on inflammatory markers and its confirmation by in-silico strategy. *Thai Journal of Pharmaceutical Sciences*, *45*(6), 532–544.

20. Segall, M. D. (2012). Multi-parameter optimization: Identifying high quality compounds with a balance of properties. *Current Pharmaceutical Design*, *18*, 1292–1310.
21. Hann, M. M., & Keseru, G. M. (2012). Finding the sweet spot: The role of nature and nurture in medicinal chemistry. *Nature Reviews Drug Discovery*, *11*, 355–365.
22. Bian, Y., & Xie, X. Q. (2021). Generative chemistry: Drug discovery with deep learning generative models. *Journal of Molecular Modeling*, *27*, 71.
23. Aminabee, S. K., Santhi Krupa, D., Hanumanth Rao, K., Sirisha, V., Anitha Kumari, V., Nagasen, D., Sujiya, B., & Leelavati, T. S. (2023). Pharmacoeconomic analysis of biologic vs. biosimilar therapies in rheumatoid arthritis. *International Journal of Chemical and Biochemical Sciences*, *24*(4), 395–400.
24. Coley, C. W., Green, W. H., & Jensen, K. F. (2018). Machine learning in computer-aided synthesis planning. *Accounts of Chemical Research*, *51*, 1281–1289.
25. Webb, D., & Jamison, T. F. (2010). Continuous flow multi-step organic synthesis. *Chemical Science*, *1*, 675–680.
26. Leelavati, T. S., Madhavi, S., Kamal, G., Raju, P. V. M., Susmitha, K., Vinod, M., & Aminabee, S. K. (2023). Revolutionizing healthcare delivery: Telemedicine's influence on access and patient satisfaction. *International Journal of Chemical and Biochemical Sciences*, *24*(5), 106–115.
27. Whitehead, T. M., Irwin, B. W. J., Hunt, P., Segall, M. D., & Conduit, G. J. (2019). Imputation of assay bioactivity data using deep learning. *Journal of Chemical Information and Modeling*, *59*, 1197–1204.
28. Irwin, B. W. J., Levell, J. R., Whitehead, T. M., Segall, M. D., & Conduit, G. J. (2020). Practical applications of deep learning to impute heterogeneous drug discovery data. *Journal of Chemical Information and Modeling*, *60*, 2848–2857.
29. Aminabee, S. K., Devi Mallika, K., & Lakshmana Rao, A. (2023). Natural resources in management and treatment of diseases: A review. *Pharma Times*, *55*(11), 7–10.
30. Dolgos, H., Trusheim, M., Gross, D., Halle, J. P., Ogden, J., & Osterwalder, B. et al (2016). Translational medicine guide transforms drug development processes: The recent Merck experience. *Drug Discovery Today*, *21*, 517–526.
31. Toh, T. S., Dondelinger, F., & Wang, D. (2019). Looking beyond the hype: Applied AI and machine learning in translational medicine. *EBioMedicine*, *47*, 607–615.
32. Ekins, S., Puhl, A. C., Zorn, K. M., Lane, T. R., Russo, D. P., & Klein, J. J. et al. (2019). Exploiting machine learning for end-to-end drug discovery and development. *Nature Materials*, *18*, 435–441.
33. Aminabee, S. K., & Lakshmana Rao, A. (2024). Computational identification of selected bioactive compounds from *Cedrus deodara* as inhibitors against SARS-CoV-2 main protease: A pharmacoinformatics study. *Indian Drugs*, *61*(2), 78–91.
34. Vamathevan, J., Clark, D., Czodrowski, P., Dunham, I., Ferran, E., & Lee, G. et al. (2019). Applications of machine learning in drug discovery and development. *Nature Reviews Drug Discovery*, *18*, 463–477.
35. Lo, Y. C., Rensi, S. E., Torng, W., & Altman, R. B. (2018). Machine learning in chemoinformatics and drug discovery. *Drug Discovery Today*, *23*, 1538–1546.
36. Zhavoronkov, A., Ivanenkov, Y. A., Aliper, A., Veselov, M. S., Aladinskiy, V. A., & Aladinskaya, A. V., et al. (2019). Deep learning enables rapid identification of potent DDR1 kinase inhibitors. *Nature Biotechnology*, *37*, 1038–1040.
37. Ravi Shankar, K., Aminabee, S. K., Ramana, G., Chenchu Lakshmi, K. N. V., & Indusree, G. (2024). Formulation and evaluation of propranolol hydrochloride floating tablets by 32 factorial design. *International Journal of Drug Delivery Technology*, *14*(4), 2060–2067.
38. Sellwood, M. A., Ahmed, M., Segler, M. H., & Brown, N. (2018). Artificial intelligence in drug discovery. *Future Medicinal Chemistry*, *10*(17), 2025–2028.

7 Regulatory Considerations and Ethical Implications

Introduction

Pharmaceutical research experienced a major transformation through computational methodologies which were implemented in drug discovery and development processes. Molecular modeling and machine learning (ML) alongside artificial intelligence (AI) and big data analytics minimized both development period and production expenses for optimizing drug candidates.

The safety and quality and efficacy of therapeutic products alongside human dignity and patient rights must always be protected by regulatory and ethical guidelines when implementing computational methods [1].

In computational drug development, compliance with regulatory standards is critical. Regulatory compliance ensures that the methods and results generated through computational tools are scientifically valid, reproducible, and acceptable for decision-making in drug approval processes. Companies need to follow guidance which addresses certain aspects, such as model validation as well as data integrity and algorithm transparency and software quality assurance procedures. Computational methods require strict compliance with data privacy statutes which combined with regulations regarding patient data care and ethical operation practices. Failure to meet these requirements can lead to setbacks in drug approval, financial losses, and reputational damage for research institutions and pharmaceutical companies alike.

The importance of ethical considerations in computational drug discovery cannot be overstated. Several ethical problems in healthcare emerge from algorithmic bias alongside the improper utilization of patient information and uninformed patient consent in data acquisition and variable technical healthcare accessibility. Inadequate representation of datasets affects algorithm training because it allows biases to form during processing which generates imprecise predictions that produce damaging or inefficient treatment plans for specific groups of patients [2]. Therefore, ethical frameworks must be implemented to promote fairness, accountability, and transparency in computational research. Additionally, clear communication with stakeholders, including patients, regulators, and healthcare providers is essential to foster trust in these emerging technologies.

The regulatory structure for computational drug discovery remains under development in various countries throughout the world. The well-defined regulatory

DOI: 10.4324/9781003616177-7

systems for traditional drug development face novel hurdles from computational approaches which approval frameworks now start to handle. The U.S. Food and Drug Administration (FDA) and the European Medicines Agency (EMA) and Pharmaceuticals and Medical Devices Agency (PMDA) in Japan started implementing computational methods into their current regulatory framework. However, differences in regional policies, technological maturity, and regulatory acceptance remain significant. Collaborative efforts, such as the International Council for Harmonisation (ICH), aim to standardize regulatory requirements across countries, but a universally accepted framework specific to computational drug development is still in development. The worldwide development of a strong regulatory environment demands continuous communication between regulators and industry stakeholders with ethicists about computational method advancement [3].

Regulatory Frameworks Governing Computational Drug Discovery

U.S. FDA Guidelines for In Silico Submissions

As a leader in drug regulation, the U.S. FDA takes the main role in merging computational models throughout its regulatory framework. The FDA recorded in silico tool potential through MIDD guidance that includes PBPK and PopPK modeling to advance development efficiency and decrease costs. The agency emphasizes transparency, reproducibility, and scientific justification in all computational submissions. Developers are expected to validate their models thoroughly, outline assumptions, and provide detailed documentation. FDA officials invite stakeholders to organize pre-submission sessions which define how computational techniques will service regulatory choices for particular applications [4].

European Medicines Agency (EMA) Perspective

The EMA supports contemporary modeling technology for drug development modernization as an integral aspect of its strategic goals. The organization leads active promotion of quantitative systems pharmacology (QSP) and both PopPK and PBPK modeling approaches. The EMA expects robust model qualification and justification, along with well-documented methodologies to ensure reproducibility and clarity. The agency has issued reflection papers and guidance documents to help applicants understand the expectations for submitting in silico data. To maintain regulatory compliance, companies should use the EMA procedures for scientific advice at the start of development to develop a common modeling strategy [5].

ICH Guidelines and Global Harmonization

The ICH stands responsible for developing worldwide standard regulations in major geographic areas. The ICH has shifted its attention from clinical and quality safety protocols to regulate the expanding utilization of computational technologies. Emerging discussions within ICH are exploring frameworks for digital tools and model-based approaches. By promoting global harmonization, ICH aims to

Table 7.1 Major Regulatory Bodies and Their Focus on Computational Drug Discovery

Regulatory Body	*Region*	*Key Focus Areas*	*Notable Guidelines/Actions*
FDA	United States	In silico submissions, AI validation, PBPK modeling	Guidance on Model-Informed Drug Development (MIDD)
EMA	Europe	Systems pharmacology, data transparency, modeling standards	EMA Reflection Paper on Modeling and Simulation
ICH	Global (Harmonization)	Standardization across member countries	ICH M12, ICH E6 (R3)
CDSCO	India	Emerging computational frameworks, preclinical regulations	Integration with AYUSH and biosimilars
PMDA	Japan	Predictive modeling, early stage simulation	Collaboration with academic and industry stakeholders

facilitate consistent evaluation of in silico evidence, reduce redundancy in regulatory review, and enable smoother international drug approvals. Modeling has become commonplace in pharmaceutical development so ICH plays an essential role to establish global standards about quality and use of these models [6].

Emerging Frameworks in Asia-Pacific and BRICS Countries

The Asia-Pacific together with BRICS regions experience swift development of regulatory systems devoted to computational drug discovery. China together with India are establishing in silico methods as part of their review procedures especially when developing biosimilars while screening drugs for toxicity effects and making pharmacokinetic predictions. China's National Medical Products Administration (NMPA) and India's Central Drugs Standard Control Organization (CDSCO) are showing increasing openness to digital innovation, often participating in international collaborations to strengthen their regulatory capacity. The governments of Singapore and South Korea are using their resources to develop regulatory science and infrastructure programs which enhance computational innovation capabilities [7]. While these frameworks are still developing, they reflect a growing commitment to adopting global best practices in computational drug development (Table 7.1).

Preclinical Data and In Silico Validation Requirements

Regulatory Acceptance of Molecular Docking and QSAR Models

The preclinical stage of computational drug discovery heavily depends on QSAR modeling together with molecular docking as its essential tools. Such methods serve dual purposes by determining drug-target interactions and calculating biological response from chemical makeup. Regulatory agencies, such as the FDA and EMA, have begun recognizing the utility of these models, provided they are supported by strong validation and scientific rationale. For regulatory acceptance, developers must demonstrate the reliability, robustness, and predictive power of the models. Usability assessments incorporate statistical verification with dedicated training and test components alongside well-defined reach areas that establish biochemical outcome dependencies from chemical features. These computational tools need regulatory approval documents that detail their contribution to the decision-making process especially for enhancing lead compounds and forecasting toxicity as well as selecting compounds for laboratory production and testing [8].

Validating Virtual Screening and Simulation Data

The combination of virtual screening and molecular simulations which include molecular dynamics (MD) functions as an effective pair for finding optimal drug candidates. Data generated through these methods needs complete validation for regulatory authorities to accept it. The evaluation process includes inspecting raw data quality and testing numerical modeling methods while compared to confirmed experimental results when applicable. Validation strategies often involve cross-validation, retrospective testing on known ligands, and comparison with biological assays. Regulators also look for reproducibility in virtual screening workflows whether similar results can be obtained using different software tools or computational setups. A comprehensive documentation of methods together with scoring functions needs to go hand in hand with performance metrics and reporting parameters in order to build credibility and ensure transparency [9]. Ultimately, while simulation data may not yet replace experimental studies, validated in silico evidence can significantly support regulatory submissions and reduce experimental burden (Table 7.2).

Reproducibility and Transparency of Computational Predictions

Regulators express primary concern about computational models because they need clear predictions which can easily be reproduced. The ability to replicate results in different laboratories and studies depends on reproducibility which allows the exact replication of study or laboratory findings. To meet regulatory expectations, all aspects of computational workflows – software versions, algorithms, parameters,

Table 7.2 Validation and Reporting Requirements for Computational Models

Aspect	*Requirement*
Model Documentation	Description of assumptions, algorithms, and parameters
Data Quality	Use of curated, peer-reviewed, or validated datasets
Reproducibility	Code availability, workflow transparency, version control
Verification & Validation	Internal testing, benchmarking, comparison with experimental data
Uncertainty Quantification	Sensitivity analysis, confidence intervals, probabilistic modeling

datasets, and hardware environments must be well-documented and accessible. Transparency also involves making the rationale behind modeling decisions clear, including how parameters were chosen and how uncertainty was handled. In recent years, there has been a growing push toward open science and standardized reporting practices in computational research. Guidelines, such as the OECD principles for QSAR validation and the FDA, require model-informed submissions to display reproducible standards because such standards promote regulatory trust. Computational predictions help generate credible evidence that becomes beneficial for preclinical drug development when these principles are properly followed [10].

Good Modeling Practices (GMP)

Standards for Computational Model Development

GMPs function as an essential definitive structure that directs computational model creation as well as evaluation and deployment within pharmaceutical discovery practice. Standardized procedures receive backing from regulatory agencies as well as scientific organizations to provide quality and dependable computational results. Standards focus on three main points for modeling which include objective definition at development time together with algorithm selection and dataset utilization in addition to scientifically based assumptions. Model developers are encouraged to adopt structured workflows that allow for consistency, traceability, and scalability. Relevant global organizations, including the FDA through their MIDD program together with the OECD have established guidelines which promote adoption of validated mechanistic models. Standards in computational practices improve both regulatory trust in results as well as student and professional collaboration [11].

Documentation and Reporting Requirements

The practice of comprehensive documentation stands essential for modeling practices when computational outcomes need to guide regulatory or clinical choices. Model reporting to regulatory bodies must demonstrate a comprehensive overview that includes descriptions about the model's reason for existence together with its design specifications and sourcing methods for datasets and details regarding development practices as well as deployment settings. A detailed compilation of software documentation involves recording all versions as well as input parameters and documented assumptions and model development reasons. Furthermore, reporting should clearly communicate the model's limitations, potential sources of bias, and scope of applicability. Standardized reporting templates together with technical documentation checklists receive greater promotion by regulatory bodies to establish consistent review operations. When models are properly documented stakeholders can reproduce results and scientific communities can analyze the work while developing trust in computational evidence [12].

Verification, Validation, and Uncertainty Quantification

A computational model requires the combination of verification, validation, and uncertainty quantification (VVUQ) techniques to generate acceptable results as well as meet its intended performance. Verification activities consist of checks to determine correct implementation of the model through error-free logical operations and error-free programming. The validation process requires an assessment between model-predicted values and experimental data to determine prediction accuracy levels. Internal validation techniques based on cross-validation methods and external assessment using separate datasets compose the evaluation process. Uncertainty quantification, however, addresses the confidence level of the model's outputs by assessing the impact of data variability, parameter assumptions, and structural uncertainties. Regulatory agencies increasingly expect VVUQ activities to be performed systematically and reported transparently, as they form the basis for assessing the credibility and reliability of computational tools in decision-making. Computational models offer decisive risk reduction power through rigorous application of VVUQ principles which guides different stages of pharmaceutical development [13].

Regulatory Submission of In Silico Evidence

Integration of Computational Data in IND/NDA Submissions

Computational methods have prompted the widespread submission of in silico information within regulatory documents, such as Investigational New Drug (IND) applications and New Drug Applications (NDA). The potential of in silico data for drug development decision support now receives approval from regulatory agencies specifically when experimental evidence is restricted or hard to obtain. In silico models can be integrated into submissions to justify dosing strategies, predict drug-drug interactions, assess organ-specific toxicity, or inform study designs. To succeed with computational integration the presented evidence requires detailed experimental results coordinated with robust scientific justification and it must also include strengthened validation along with complete documentation. Sponsors can obtain clear directions from the FDA regarding regulatory approval expectations for their model use through early meetings before submitting the Investigational New Drug (IND) application [14].

Use of PBPK and QSP Models in Regulatory Dossiers

In silico regulatory dossiers accept PBPK and QSP models as their two main accepted modeling techniques. The ability of PBPK models to use physiological parameters and simulate drug distribution along with absorption and metabolism together with excretion makes them effective for special population pharmacokinetic predictions, such as pediatrics and geriatrics and hepatorenal impaired patients. QSP models go a step further by integrating biological pathways and disease mechanisms to predict drug efficacy and safety at the systems level. Regulatory agencies have accepted PBPK models for label expansion, bridging studies, and evaluating drug-drug interactions. QSP models serve as relatively recent additions to regulatory applications because they demonstrate value through their mechanistic capabilities and decision-making support in clinical trial development. The whole scientific authority of regulatory dossiers receives enhancement from submitting model types accompanied by detailed methodology and simulation results and validation information [15].

Case Studies of Regulatory-Approved In Silico Evidence

Multiple regulatory submissions have proven the effectiveness of in silico evidence for achieving approvals through case study demonstrations. The FDA has accepted PBPK modeling in numerous applications to create pediatric dosing recommendations that do not warrant extra clinical trials. In one prominent case, PBPK models enabled the FDA to approve label modifications for a pediatric antifungal drug based on simulated exposure levels. Similarly, QSP models have been employed in oncology and immunology to predict treatment responses and optimize combination therapy regimens. Virtual bioequivalence studies as well as exposure predictions for drugs with complex delivery systems now find acceptance through regulatory agencies, including EMA together with other international regulatory bodies. The acceptance of computational data by regulators continues to grow because they trust properly developed and validated models that maintain transparency in their publication [16]. They also demonstrate the evolving role of in silico tools as not just supportive, but sometimes pivotal, elements in regulatory decision-making (Figure 7.1).

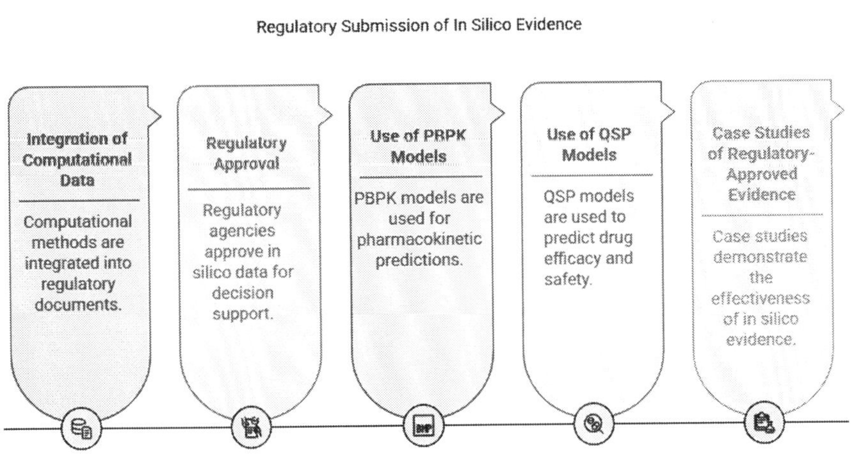

Figure 7.1 Regulatory Submission of In Silico Evidence

Artificial Intelligence and Machine Learning in Regulatory Context

Regulatory Readiness of AI-Based Predictions

The drug discovery and development field experiences rapid transformation through AI and ML technology which brings strong capabilities to pattern recognition and predictive modeling and automated processes. The process of submitting AI predictions to regulators requires unique considerations because of specific challenges. The three factors responsible for AI model regulatory readiness are transparency coupled with robustness and reproducibility. Agencies, such as the U.S. FDA and EMA, are actively exploring frameworks to evaluate AI tools, focusing on the validity and context of use. For AI-based predictions to be accepted, developers must demonstrate the quality of input data, the rationale behind model selection, and the interpretability of outcomes. The FDA presents an updated regulatory system for AI/ML-based Software as a Medical Device (SaMD) through lifecycle oversight and performance monitoring and continuous learning procedures. Healthcare authorities require strict evidence analysis and validation to accept AI tools for their regulatory decision-making procedures [17].

Explainability and Bias Mitigation in AI Models

The regulatory evaluation of AI models requires comprehensive examine of their explainability capabilities since this capacity determines how well the model can reveal its prediction or decision-making processes. Rating algorithms that exhibit high accuracy face challenges because they remain nonexplainable which weakens belief in their eligibility for essential regulatory decisions. To address this, explainable AI (XAI) techniques are being developed that allow stakeholders to trace model logic and assess the influence of various inputs. Moreover, bias mitigation is essential to ensure that AI models do not propagate or amplify existing disparities in drug response or patient outcomes. A growing regulatory requirement for developers includes conducting audits to show how they identified and detected bias alongside their methods of reducing bias during model development. The implementation of AI tools in healthcare and drug development depends on available data reporting along with training methods and validation protocols and population statistics to maintain equal and scientific valid applications [18].

GxP Compliance for AI-Driven Tools

AI tools need to respect Good Practice standards based on their use and function as Good Clinical Practice (GCP), Good Laboratory Practice (GLP) and Good Manufacturing Practice (GMP) to operate within regulated domains. Systems achieve GxP compliance through measures which guarantee their reliability and trackability and security when they help with regulatory decisions or product quality assessments. AI models must be developed and deployed under validated systems, with rigorous documentation, audit trails, and version control. Additionally, change management procedures must be in place to handle model updates or retraining, particularly for adaptive AI systems that evolve with new data. Regulatory bodies are establishing requirements for AI tools under GxP compliance which includes validation together with risk assessment and governance requirements. Sponsors who develop AI systems according to GxP principles will improve acceptance by regulators for their digital solutions throughout drug discovery processes and beyond [19].

Ethical Considerations in In Silico Drug Discovery

Algorithmic Transparency and Bias

ML algorithms coupled with AI systems have become essential for drug discovery but the ethical issues concerning algorithm visibility and prejudice are increasing. The ability to understand how predictive models reach their outputs is known as Algorithmic transparency while this transparency ensures fairness and reproduces decisions and holds people accountable. In drug discovery, biased algorithms could lead to skewed predictions, potentially resulting in harmful outcomes, especially if certain demographic groups are underrepresented in the data. For instance, biased models could affect the identification of drug candidates that may not work effectively for certain populations [20]. The framework of ethical practices for in silico drug discovery requires complete documentation of model architecture as well as dataset selection and algorithmic decision-making pathways. The trust of regulatory authorities and researchers and patients depends on maintaining explainabilty and auditable capabilities in AI tools for reducing bias.

Data Privacy and Ownership Issues

The implementation of expansive data collections in computerized drug discovery with AI and ML technologies creates substantial moral dilemmas about personal information security and database rights. The models operating in a virtual environment depend on extensive datasets that might contain protected patient information as well as genomic data and proprietary scientific knowledge. Data security control stands among the highest priorities. Ethical guidelines require that data be anonymized, encrypted, and used in compliance with data protection regulations, such as the General Data Protection Regulation (GDPR) in Europe or the Health Insurance Portability and Accountability Act (HIPAA) in the U.S. Furthermore, ownership of data particularly data collected from clinical trials or genomics research must be clearly defined [21]. Ethical issues emerge because the goals of data providers, including patients and researchers from institutions differ from those of pharmaceutical enterprises and technology development teams. The proper implementation of in silico drug discovery requires respecting patient rights by ensuring data privacy and attaining informed consent and maintaining open transparency in data sharing practices. This framework will protect individual rights and respect ethical standards (Figure 7.2).

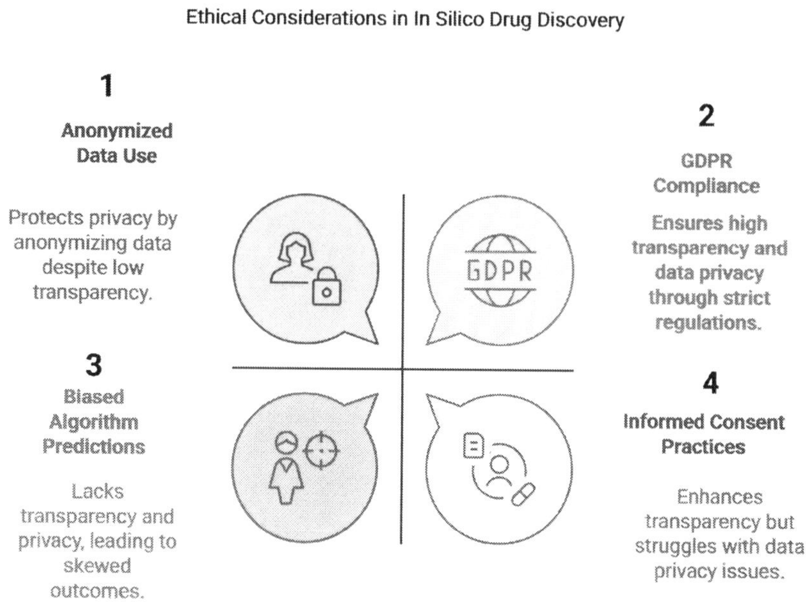

Figure 7.2 Ethical Considerations in In Silico Drug Discovery

Ethical Use of AI in Personalized Medicine and Genomics

In silico and AI techniques create essential building blocks for personalized medicine because they help doctors provide treatments matched to genomic profiles combined with biological details of individual patients. The proper utilization of AI technology in personalized medicine and genomics management touches multiple significant ethical challenges. The main problem with genetic information-based discrimination is its ability to restrict treatment access as well as insurance coverage and professional career options. Ethical guidelines must ensure that AI models used in personalized medicine are developed with careful consideration of equity, inclusivity, and fairness. Moreover, as genomic data becomes more central to drug discovery, it is essential to address the implications of genetic privacy and consent [22]. Patients and individuals providing genomic information must be fully informed of how their data will be used and the potential risks of its misuse. The use of ethical principles needs to regulate AI applications in genomics to advance science and defend the rights of humanity concerning privacy and freedom and personal dignity.

Intellectual Property and Data Protection

Patentability of AI-Designed Molecules

The invention of AI together with ML techniques in pharmaceutical discovery creates core patentability issues for molecules created through AI processes. Patent regulations throughout time have centered their attention on human creativity together with inventor roles yet the creation of AI-generated molecules requires a review of this system. The main problem resides in determining whether AI deserves the title of "inventor" or if the patent should be assigned to researchers and organizations responsible for AI system development. Legal scholars and patent offices are debating how to address these challenges. Some jurisdictions, like the U.S. and Europe, have begun to recognize AI's role in the invention process, but they still require a human inventor to be listed. AI-designed molecules face additional legal considerations regarding their patentability because novelty together with non-obviousness and utility functions as essential patent approval criteria [23]. The patent systems face challenges to evolve when addressing new AI-driven drug design technologies because they must reconcile the rights of pharmaceutical companies with those of AI developers and patent systems.

Ownership of AI-Generated Discoveries

Intelligent IP systems need to reconcile multiple priorities between ownership rights for discoveries created through AI technology. AI systems that automatically create drug candidates or solutions have no defined owner of their innovation rights. The dimensions of decision-making in this situation extend to AI developers who developed the algorithms as well as the entities that supplied training data alongside the pharmaceutical companies backing the scientific research. The absence of clear intellectual property rights makes disputes possible which then delays the process of treatment development and commercialization. Legal frameworks are gradually evolving to address these questions, but the issue remains unresolved in many jurisdictions [24]. The ownership of AI-generated discoveries must be carefully negotiated through contracts, intellectual property agreements, and licensing deals to ensure fair compensation and incentives for all parties involved. The progression of AI toward central innovation requires firm legal stipulations that will defend both AI systems and their developers alongside researchers and stakeholders of industry.

Regulatory and Legal Aspects of Data Sharing

Scientific research expansion heavily relies on data sharing especially within computational drug discovery where various datasets connect to boosting AI model prediction abilities. The regulatory framework together with the applicable legal aspects make data sharing processes challenging to operate. Data protection laws, such as GDPR in Europe and HIPAA in the U.S., regulate how personal and sensitive data must be handled, stored, and shared. In drug discovery, the sharing of clinical trial data, patient records, or genomic data for AI training models must comply with these privacy laws to ensure that individuals' rights are protected. Intellectual property issues create barriers for organizations when it comes to data sharing because they need to establish proper legal safeguards before disclosing proprietary datasets. The rise of data sharing activities features initiatives dedicated to protecting ethics alongside transparency in such sharing along with secure implementation of data platforms which address open science alongside privacy management and commercial requirements [25]. Several regulatory bodies have started providing rules about trial data dissemination in addition to creating secure environments where researchers can work together while maintaining data security.

Digital Clinical Trials and Virtual Patients

Regulatory Status of Digital Twin Models

Clinical research as well as drug development welcomes the rising utilization of patient-specific and system-specific digital twin models that function as virtual duplicates of real-world products and individuals. The simulation models analyze present and past clinical data to produce virtual representations of patient bodily functions and disease path and drug response outcomes which enable drug testing before human testing. However, the regulatory status of digital twin models is still evolving. Regulatory bodies like the U.S. FDA and EMA are cautiously optimistic but demand high levels of scientific rigor, validation, and transparency before considering digital twins for decision-making. Research activities involving digital twins take place in three areas, including preclinical trials and pharmacokinetic modeling and personalized dosing assessment [26]. The regulatory authorities must receive thorough documentation about development procedures and data origins while knowing how the predictions match clinical results alongside prediction boundary definitions. While not yet a mainstream regulatory tool, digital twins are positioned to become integral components of digital clinical trials, provided that standards for their qualification and use are clearly established (Table 7.3).

Ethical Oversight in AI-Simulated Clinical Trials

Evaluations carried out with AI-simulated clinical trials demonstrate promise to significantly cut costs and minimize both trial duration and moral responsibility issues which standard human clinical investigations usually experience. In silico

Table 7.3 Use of AI Models in Regulatory Submissions – Readiness Spectrum

AI Application	*Regulatory Readiness*	*Use Case Example*	*Challenges*
Predictive Toxicology	Moderate	Early filtering of toxic compounds	Limited validation datasets
Image-Based Drug Screening	Low to Moderate	Deep learning on microscopy/ pathology images	Explainability, generalizability
PBPK/Systems Modeling	High	Dose optimization, pediatric drug development	Complex model validation
AI in Clinical Trial Design	Emerging	Enrollment prediction, endpoint selection	Ethical and patient diversity concerns

models enable the simulation of patient conduct and disease progression as well as drug response assessment which sometimes takes the place of or supports select trial steps. The new innovation introduces substantial moral dilemmas. Missing real human participants in simulated experiments can result in unnoticed biases or inaccurate modeling outcomes because such flaws might cause severe issues when used by clinicians for diagnostic purposes. Ethical oversight in AI-simulated trials should ensure that models are based on high-quality, representative data, and that their predictions are independently validated [27]. These assessments from regulatory and ethical bodies need to define how simulations should be used as either exploratory or confirmatory tests before establishing their acceptable result-interpreting thresholds. Just like conventional trials, AI-driven trials must undergo ethical review to ensure scientific integrity, risk management, and the responsible use of digital technologies.

Consent and Risk Communication in Virtual Environments

Patients participating in digital clinical trials with virtual participants and remote monitoring systems need to receive different types of informed consent and risk communication information. Participants need complete knowledge about the utilization of their data and analysis methods as well as storage methods along with the functions of all AI and digital research platforms involved in the process. The electronic procedure for obtaining consent must contain reliable authentication methods to demonstrate participants have full comprehension while freely participating in trials. Additionally, communicating potential risks, such as data breaches, algorithmic errors, or limitations in predictive accuracy, must be done in clear and accessible language. Researchers and sponsors are ethically obligated to ensure transparency, data security, and continuous communication with participants throughout the trial. Regulatory agencies now issue guidance documents about electronic informed consent (eIC) along with digital engagement best practices because they aim to preserve traditional in-person trial ethical requirements in new digital trial frameworks [28].

Open Science vs. Proprietary Tools

Open-Source Tools and Their Regulatory Implications

The discovery process for new drugs significantly benefits from open-source tools because these platforms provide accessible systems for modeling and simulation and data analysis. The scientific research gains transparency and broad collaboration together with result reproducibility through these enabling tools that support innovation. Using these tools in regulatory submission processes requires special attention to multiple key points. The FDA and EMA together with other regulatory authorities demand proper documentation and validation of tools that they authorize for use whether open-source or proprietary in nature. Open-source software must demonstrate reliability, traceability, and consistency, especially if used to support clinical or pharmacological claims [29]. Developers are expected to provide detailed documentation, version control history, and evidence of peer review or community validation. To gain regulatory dossier acceptance and credibility open tools must pass strict quality tests. Regulatory bodies evaluate open-source tools because they must verify that their open nature does not threaten scientific precision and protect research data reliability.

Transparency vs. Commercial Interests in Drug Modeling

The main conflict in computational drug development emerges from the need to protect business secrets while maintaining scientific visibility. Open science promotes collaborative model sharing and algorithm distribution and data exchange, thus facilitating scientific monitoring and teamwork. Proprietary tools require substantial investment and companies tightly control their ownership to defend against competitors. This dichotomy can create conflicts during regulatory evaluation, where transparency is essential for assessing the validity and reliability of computational models. Regulators need pharmaceutical companies to provide thorough descriptions of proprietary system operations but these companies often hesitate to share detailed information despite regulatory requirements [30]. Navigating this tension requires a strategic approach that respects intellectual property while fulfilling regulatory expectations for accountability and reproducibility. Increasingly, hybrid models are being adopted where core methodologies are shared openly, while specific applications or datasets remain protected helping bridge the gap between innovation and regulation (Table 7.4).

FAIR Data Principles in Regulatory Submissions

The FAIR data principles include Findability, Accessibility, Interoperability, and Reusability which create an effective framework to ensure transparent and efficient research data management. When applied in regulatory data submissions for computational drug discovery FAIR principles increase the value along with credibility of the data. FAIR data alignment enables regulatory bodies to both identify data origins and validate results in addition to providing them access to reuse information during later assessments. Moreover, adherence to FAIR principles

Table 7.4 Comparison – Open-Source vs. Proprietary Computational Tools

Feature	*Open-Source Tools*	*Proprietary Tools*
Accessibility	Freely available	Subscription or licensing fees required
Transparency	High (source code open for review)	Low (protected algorithms and logic)
Customization	Easily customizable	Limited flexibility
Regulatory Acceptance	Requires documentation and validation	Often includes pre-approved validation modules
IP Protection	Minimal	Strong IP protection

aligns with global movements toward data openness and scientific collaboration, without necessarily compromising proprietary interests. Regulatory bodies are increasingly encouraging or requiring the use of standardized data formats and metadata descriptions to facilitate review processes. Renewed regulation becomes more efficient when research teams adopt FAIR practices alongside sponsors which helps produce an improved transparent scientific environment. Different jurisdictions need to address the harmonization challenges for FAIR implementation specifically regarding the combined use of proprietary and open data under one framework [4].

Future Directions in Regulatory Science

Regulatory Sandboxes for Digital Health Innovation

The fast evolution of drug development technology and digital healthcare requires regulatory bodies to establish regulatory sandboxes for supporting rapid progression. Such controlled environments give researchers and companies the chance to evaluate new diagnostic tools and digital disease treatments along with virtual clinical testing platforms in close partnership with regulators yet without complete requirement to follow rules. Regulatory sandboxes encourage innovation while maintaining oversight and public safety, allowing regulators to better understand emerging technologies and shape appropriate guidelines. For computational drug discovery, sandboxes could facilitate the real-time evaluation of AI models, virtual patient platforms, or novel data integration methods [31]. The sandboxes create a proactive approach that enables regulatory science transformation for future-ready paradigms through better dialogue between innovators and regulators to speed up secure implementation of new healthcare tools.

Role of Real-World Evidence and Computational Epidemiology

The growing importance of real-world evidence (RWE) which emerges from electronic health records and insurance claims together with patient registries has become essential for regulatory decisions. RWE becomes a strong evaluation method for assessing drug safety and effectiveness alongside usage patterns for different populations by combining it with computational tools. Computational epidemiology extends this concept further by using models and simulations to understand disease spread, treatment outcomes, and public health dynamics at scale. These approaches allow regulators to make informed, timely decisions that reflect actual healthcare practices and population-level impacts. Regulatory bodies are presently working on integrating RWE with computational epidemiology despite their evolving implementation pathway since this combination demonstrates potential for filling gaps in traditional trials. All these tools show potential to become essential components of regulatory science after the healthcare data infrastructure enhancements together with the resolution of privacy issues [32].

Evolving Standards for AI, Big Data, and Quantum Computing

The advancement of biomedical research along with drug discovery through AI, big data and quantum computing requires regulatory science to develop specific standards to authorize their proper utilization. AI models that use deep learning require ongoing validation and performance tests to guarantee their accuracy and interpretability without favoritism. Analytics of big data presents multiple operational difficulties concerning heterogeneous sources and varied origins and compatibility between systems that require comprehensive data management standards. However the current stage of progress in quantum computing holds revolutionary implications for handling difficult molecular modeling along with optimization tasks for drug creation processes. Regulators must begin preparing for the implications of quantum technologies by collaborating with experts and drafting preliminary guidance [33]. Globally standardized advanced technology standards which look forward need to be established to ensure proper integration of innovative systems into medical development cycles and healthcare environments.

Conclusion

Balancing Innovation with Oversight

Drug discovery speed, cost effectiveness and accuracy level have increased significantly through computational technology implementation in drug development. The new innovation requires thorough regulatory protection that safeguards both safety performance and ethical standards of therapeutic products. Widespread global regulatory bodies now update their guidelines through collaborative initiatives along with implementing new approaches that include regulatory sandboxes. As the use of AI, in silico models, and digital platforms becomes more widespread, it is essential that these tools are subjected to rigorous validation, documentation, and ethical scrutiny. Drugs of the future will develop through technological enhancements while humanity ensures proper management of this innovative process [34].

Toward Ethical, Compliant, and Transparent Drug Discovery

Computational drug discovery must look toward the future by establishing ethical practices as well as regulatory requirements and scientific openness as fundamental principles. Ensuring algorithmic fairness, protecting data privacy, and fostering open collaboration are crucial to building trust in digital methodologies. Compliance with global regulatory frameworks, adherence to GMPs, and incorporation of FAIR data principles will strengthen the credibility of computational evidence in regulatory submissions. A society-wide ecosystem emerges when stakeholders unify cultural advancement with legal parameters, thus creating a safe environment that promotes scientific innovation together with public health protection [35].

References

1. Grote, T., & Berens, P. (2020). On the ethics of algorithmic decision-making in healthcare. *Journal of Medical Ethics*, *46*(3), 205–211.
2. Aminabee, S. K., Prabhakar, M. C., Prasad, R. G. S. V., & Lakshmana Rao, A. (2011). Screening the pharmacological activity of cerium oxide nanoparticles in-vitro. *Biomedical and Pharmacology Journal*, *4*(2), 287–289.
3. Magrabi, F., Ammenwerth, E., McNair, J. B., De Keizer, N. F., Hyppönen, H., Nykänen, P., Rigby, M., Scott, P. J., Vehko, T., & Wong, Z. S.-Y., et al. (2019). Artificial intelligence in clinical decision support: Challenges for evaluating AI and practical implications. *Yearbook of Medical Informatics*, *28*, 128–134.
4. Kumar, Y., Koul, A., Singla, R., & Ijaz, M. F. (2022). Artificial intelligence in disease diagnosis: A systematic literature review, synthesizing framework and future research agenda. *Journal of Ambient Intelligence and Humanized Computing*, *14*(7), 1–28.
5. Aminabee, S. K., Lakshmana Rao, A., Sowmya, K., Nymisha, D., Kusuma Naga Lakshmi, K., Manikanta, K. V. N. S., & Praveen Kumar, P. (2019). Evaluation of analgesic activity of *Ficus palmata*. *Iranian Journal of Pharmaceutical Sciences*, *15*(3), 47–60.
6. Vulli, A., Srinivasu, P. N., Sashank, M. S. K., Shafi, J., Choi, J., & Ijaz, M. F. (2022). Fine-tuned DenseNet-169 for breast cancer metastasis prediction using fastai and 1-cycle policy. *Sensors*, *22*, 2988.
7. Aminabee, S. K., Lakshmana Rao, A., & Chinna Eswaraiah, M. (2020). In-vivo antioxidant activity of different fractions of *Indigofera barberi* against paracetamol-induced toxicity in rats. *Turkish Journal of Pharmaceutical Sciences*, *17*(2), 136–140.
8. Ahmad, A., Merla, F., Ali, B., Shah, A. A., AlZubi, M. A., & AlZubi, M. (2023). A deep transfer learning approach for COVID-19 detection and exploring a sense of belonging with diabetes. *Frontiers in Public Health*, *6*, 11.
9. Prasanth, D. S. N. B. K., Aminabee, S. K., Lakshmana Rao, A., Teja, N., Bhargavi, K., Monika, C., Pujitha, B., Sandhya, T., Lalitha, A., & Siva Prasad, P. (2020). Anthelmintic activity of *Mansoa alliacea* against *Pheretima posthuma*: In-vitro and in-silico approach. *Thai Journal of Pharmaceutical Sciences*, *4*(3), 186–196.
10. Kumar, M., Verma, S., Kumar, A., Ijaz, M. F., & Rawat, D. B., et al. (2022). ANAF-IoMT: A novel architectural framework for IoMT-enabled smart healthcare system by enhancing security based on RECC-VC. *IEEE Transactions on Industrial Informatics*, *18*, 8936–8943.
11. Prasanth, D. S. N. B. K., Aminabee, S. K., Lakshmana Rao, A., Guntupalli, C., Reddy, A. R., Kulandaivelu, U., Rao, S. N. K., & Rajeshwari, P. (2021). Inhibitory effects of *Mansoa alliacea* in Freund's adjuvant arthritis on inflammatory markers and its confirmation by in-silico strategy. *Thai Journal of Pharmaceutical Sciences*, *45*(6), 532–544.
12. Slavin, R. E. (1995). Best evidence synthesis: An intelligent alternative to meta-analysis. *Journal of Clinical Epidemiology*, *48*, 9–18.
13. McCarthy, J., Minsky, M. L., Rochester, N., & Shannon, C. E. (2006). A proposal for the Dartmouth summer research project on artificial intelligence, August 31, 1955. *AI Magazine*, *27*, 12–14.
14. Aminabee, S. K., Santhi Krupa, D., Hanumanth Rao, K., Sirisha, V., Anitha Kumari, V., Nagasen, D., Sujiya, B., & Leelavati, T. S. (2023). Pharmacoeconomic analysis of biologic vs. biosimilar therapies in rheumatoid arthritis. *International Journal of Chemical and Biochemical Sciences*, *24*(4), 395–400.
15. Bengio, Y., Courville, A., & Vincent, P. (2013). Representation learning: A review and new perspectives. *IEEE Transactions on Pattern Analysis and Machine Intelligence*, *35*(8), 1798–1828.
16. Leelavati, T. S., Madhavi, S., Kamal, G., Raju, P. V. M., Susmitha, K., Vinod, M., & Aminabee, S. K. (2023). Revolutionizing healthcare delivery: Telemedicine's influence on access and patient satisfaction. *International Journal of Chemical and Biochemical Sciences*, *24*(5), 106–115.

17. Schmidhuber, J. (2015). Deep learning in neural networks: An overview. *Neural Networks*, *61*, 85–117.
18. Aminabee, S. K., Devi Mallika, K., & Lakshmana Rao, A. (2023). Natural resources in management and treatment of diseases: A review. *Pharma Times*, *55*(11), 7–10.
19. Organisation for Economic Co-operation and Development. (2019). *Recommendation of the Council on Artificial Intelligence* (OECD Legal Instruments. OECD/LEGAL/0449).
20. La Vattiata, F. C. (2022). AI-based medical devices: The applicable law in the European Union. *BioLaw Journal – Rivista di BioDiritto*, *4*, 412–437.
21. Liu, R., Wang, M., Zheng, T., Zhang, R., Li, N., Chen, Z., Yan, H., & Shi, Q. (2022). An artificial intelligence-based risk prediction model of myocardial infarction. *BMC Bioinformatics*, *23*, 1–17.
22. Lambercy, O., Lehner, R., Chua, K., Wee, S. K., Rajeswaran, D. K., Kuah, C. W. K., Ang, W. T., Liang, P., Campolo, D., & Hussain, A., et al. (2021). Neurorehabilitation from a distance: Can intelligent technology support decentralized access to quality therapy? *Frontiers in Robotics and AI*, *8*, 612415.
23. Mennella, C., Maniscalco, U., De Pietro, G., & Esposito, M. (2023). The role of artificial intelligence in future rehabilitation services: A systematic literature review. *IEEE Access, 1*(1), 99.
24. Aminabee, S. K., & Lakshmana Rao, A. (2024). Computational identification of selected bioactive compounds from *Cedrus deodara* as inhibitors against SARS-CoV-2 main protease: A pharmacoinformatics study. *Indian Drugs*, *61*(2), 78–91.
25. Babic, B., Gerke, S., Evgeniou, T., & Cohen, I. G. (2021). Beware explanations from AI in health care. *Science*, *373*(6552), 284–286.
26. Layman, E. J. (2008). Ethical issues and the electronic health record. *Health Care Manager*, *27*(2), 165–176.
27. Braun, M., Hummel, P., Beck, S., & Dabrock, P. (2021). Primer on an ethics of AI-based decision support systems in the clinic. *Journal of Medical Ethics*, *47*(3), E3.
28. Liaw, S.-T., Powell-Davies, G., Pearce, C., Britt, H., McGlynn, L., & Harris, M. F. (2016). Optimising the use of observational electronic health record data: Current issues, evolving opportunities, strategies and scope for collaboration. *Australian Family Physician*, *45*(3), 153–156.
29. Gamble, A. (2020). Artificial intelligence and mobile apps for mental healthcare: A social informatics perspective. *Aslib Journal of Information Management*, *72*, 509–523.
30. Ravi Shankar, K., Aminabee, S. K., Ramana, G., Chenchu Lakshmi, K. N. V., & Indusree, G. (2024). Formulation and evaluation of propranolol hydrochloride floating tablets by 3^2 factorial design. *International Journal of Drug Delivery Technology*, *14*(4), 2060–2067.
31. Ghosh, P. (2018). AI early diagnosis could save heart and cancer patients. *BBC News*.
32. Lin, S. Y., Mahoney, M. R., & Sinsky, C. A. (2019). Ten ways artificial intelligence will transform primary care. *Journal of General Internal Medicine*, *34*(8), 1626–1630.
33. Esteva, A., Kuprel, B., Novoa, R. A., Ko, J., Swetter, S. M., Blau, H. M., & Thrun, S. (2017). Dermatologist-level classification of skin cancer with deep neural networks. *Nature*, *542*(7639), 115–118.
34. Guo, G. N., Jonnagaddala, J., Farshid, S., Huser, V., Reich, C., & Liaw, S.-T. (2019). Comparison of the cohort selection performance of Australian medicines terminology to anatomical therapeutic chemical mappings. *Journal of the American Medical Informatics Association*, *26*(11), 1237–1246.
35. Prasser, F., Spengler, H., Bild, R., Eicher, J., & Kuhn, K. A. (2019). Privacy-enhancing ETL-processes for biomedical data. *International Journal of Medical Informatics*, *126*, 72–81.

8 Case Studies of AI in Drug Discovery

Introduction: Unveiling the Role of AI in Drug Discovery

Evolution of Artificial Intelligence in Drug Discovery

The evolution of Artificial Intelligence (AI) in drug development started with basic automated computation yet progressed into self-governing information-based choices. Scientists initiated the implementation of rule-based algorithms and statistical models to analyze compounds as they started forecasting biological activity during the early 2000s. AI tools developed simultaneously during the time when data resources increased due to the Human Genome Project and high-throughput screening (HTS) platforms. The last decade has witnessed a rapid acceleration in AI adoption, propelled by improved computational power, open-access databases, and a surge in interest from both academia and the pharmaceutical industry. AI implements services spanning the entire drug discovery process, including both drug target assessment and lead compound enhancement as well as substance toxicity evaluation (Table 8.1).

Role of Machine Learning, Deep Learning, and NLP

Machine learning (ML) operates as the core technology behind current AI solutions in pharmaceutical discovery. ML algorithms of supervised and unsupervised categories assist scientists in identifying molecular patterns and predicting drug

Table 8.1 Evolution of AI Technologies in Drug Discovery

Era	*Key Technologies*	*Applications*	*Milestones*
Early 2000s	Rule-based Systems	Virtual screening	Limited use of AI
2010–2015	Machine Learning	QSAR modeling, docking	PubChem, ChEMBL expansion
2015–2020	Deep Learning, NLP	Target ID, synthesis prediction	AlphaFold, DeepChem
2020–Present	Generative AI, Reinforcement Learning	End-to-end drug design	ChatGPT integration, BioGPT

DOI: 10.4324/9781003616177-8

interactions and understanding how drugs affect the body. Three common ML algorithms, such as support vector machines (SVMs), random forests, and gradient boosting methods, are frequently implemented to predict bioactivity or filter chemical libraries. Deep learning (DL), a subset of ML, leverages multi-layer neural networks to understand complex biological systems. Convolutional neural networks (CNNs) are used to analyze images from high-content screening, while recurrent neural networks (RNNs) and transformers facilitate sequence analysis and molecular generation [1].

The technology of Natural Language Processing (NLP) extracts valuable information through automated processes from enormous unstructured datasets which include scientific papers, patents and both clinical trial information and electronic health records (EHRs). The usage of NLP algorithms continues to increase for discovery of new drug-disease relationships and knowledge synthesis and decision-making assistance in early drug development.

Key Milestones in AI-Driven Drug Discovery

The increasing impact of AI becomes clearer with its recent important achievements. AlphaFold by DeepMind represents a notable achievement because it made a significant advance in protein structure prediction accuracy which used to be thought impossible for decades. The AI platform Chemistry42 from Insilico Medicine producer entirely new chemical compounds at fast speeds and sent some compounds toward clinical stages. AI-based repurposing efforts during the COVID-19 pandemic, such as BenevolentAI identifying baricitinib as a potential treatment, have also demonstrated the agility and utility of AI in urgent healthcare challenges [2].

Today, AI functions beyond academic pursuits to serve as the main force behind pharmaceutical commercial activities. The pharmaceutical market witnesses numerous AI-developed candidates advancing through clinical trials, while big pharmaceutical corporations engage in AI startup partnerships to extract these innovative technologies.

Future Outlook and Opportunities

The combination of AI with future technologies that include quantum computing digital twins synthetic biology and CRISPR-based gene editing will develop advanced drug development systems. The future of precision medicine will be reshaped through AI because this technology will develop customized treatments by processing genetic information together with phenotypic and behavioral data.

However, several challenges remain. There is a pressing need for better explainability of AI models (especially black-box systems), stronger regulatory frameworks, and ethical guidelines for data use and model deployment. Combining efforts between computational scientists, clinicians, pharmacologists, and regulators will determine AI's effectiveness as a responsible instrument for drug discovery operations [3].

Methodological Framework for AI Implementation

Data Sourcing and Curation Strategies

Any AI-powered drug discovery program depends entirely on using data in its best quality and maximum volume and most relevant character. Drug research data contains molecular structures as well as protein sequences with bioactivity profiles alongside genomics and transcriptomics and proteomics information and pharmacokinetic data and clinical trial results and statements derived from EHRs.

Sourcing data requires integration from diverse repositories, such as PubChem, ChEMBL, DrugBank, PDB, and BindingDB, as well as proprietary databases within pharmaceutical companies. Raw datasets include multiple problems due to inconsistent values and missing data points as well as repeated entries. The process of data curation requires standardized molecular representation through SMILES notation alongside normalization techniques and duplicate elimination and susceptibility resolution and proper annotation of datasets for supervised learning applications [4].

Additionally, ethical considerations, such as data privacy, especially for patient-specific datasets, and compliance with regulations like GDPR and HIPAA, must be addressed during data acquisition and management.

Model Selection and Training Approaches

The foundation of successful AI deployment consists of selecting proper models after developing a curated dataset. The model selection depends on the problem type because it can be used for either classification or regression applications or clustering operations or generative modeling tasks.

- For predictive modeling (e.g., bioactivity prediction or ADMET profiling), algorithms like Random Forests, SVMs, or Gradient Boosting Machines (GBMs) are commonly used for their interpretability and performance.
- The prediction of molecular properties together with de novo molecule generation benefits from DL systems, including Graph Neural Networks (GNNs), Autoencoders and Generative Adversarial Networks (GANs), and transformer-based frameworks.
- Transfer learning and multi-task learning strategies are also gaining traction, especially when working with limited domain-specific data. These techniques allow models trained on large datasets to be fine-tuned for narrower, specific tasks in drug discovery.

A training paradigm requires the definition of suitable loss functions which includes optimizations of hyperparameters while managing unbalanced classes and uses regularization and dropout mechanisms to reduce overfitting. Model interpretability remains a critical field of study for safety reasons when DL systems operate in important biomedical Applications [5].

Validation and Optimization Techniques

Validating an AI model ensures its generalizability and reliability in unseen scenarios. Cross-validation, particularly k-fold cross-validation, is a standard approach to assess the robustness of models. Accuracy, precision, recall and F1-score, ROC-AUC and mean squared error are among the metrics that are chosen according to task type (classification or regression model).

External validation using independent datasets is critical to confirm that the model has not overfit the training data. In the pharmaceutical context, experimental validation of AI predictions, such as in vitro or in vivo studies, is also a key translational step.

Model performance reaches its best level through the application of optimization approaches which include Bayesian optimization and grid search and random search. When multiple models work together as an ensemble learning method the accuracy improves and variance decreases (Table 8.2).

Finally, for real-world deployment, models must be scalable, robust to noisy inputs, and integrated into existing bioinformatics pipelines or drug development platforms. This often necessitates collaboration with software engineers and domain scientists to build user-friendly interfaces and APIs [6].

AI in Target Identification

Drug discovery begins with precise identification of therapeutic targets that mostly involve proteins and genes or pathways which contribute to disease pathology. Rapid recognition of previously unknown targets and existing hypothesis validation are now possible because of AI innovation during this research phase. By integrating vast datasets from genomics, proteomics, transcriptomics, and biomedical literature, AI models offer unprecedented precision and scalability in uncovering disease mechanisms and pinpointing actionable targets.

Case Study 1: AI-Based Identification of Novel Kinase Targets

The functional signaling of cells depends on protein kinases because these enzymes participate extensively in diseases, including cancer. The discovery of kinase targets through traditional methods requires time-intensive experiments connected to

Table 8.2 AI Methodological Framework in Drug Discovery

Step	*Method*	*Description*	*Example Tools*
Data Sourcing	Omics, literature mining	Collection of raw data	PubMed, DrugBank
Curation	Data preprocessing	Noise removal, normalization	KNIME, Pandas
Model Selection	ML/DL algorithms	Choosing best model	XGBoost, CNN, GNN
Validation	Cross-validation, ROC	Model testing	Scikit-learn, TensorBoard

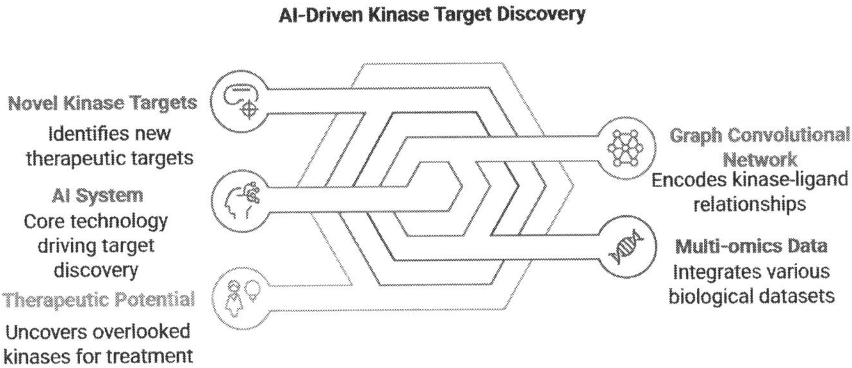

Figure 8.1 AI-Driven Kinase Target Discovery

biochemistry research alongside literature evaluation that may cause researchers to miss crucial targets. In this case study, a leading pharmaceutical company employed a DL model trained on multi-omics data, structural kinase databases, and known ligand interactions to predict novel, druggable kinase targets for oncology indications [7].

A GCN built the model by processing kinase-ligand structural information through its network and adding tumor biopsy transcriptomic data as an input. The research team demonstrated that AI identified multiple neglected kinases which showed clinical applicability in particular cancer subtypes and were experimentally validated afterward. This approach not only reduced the time to target discovery but also uncovered non-canonical kinases with therapeutic potential that had been previously overlooked (Figure 8.1).

Case Study 2: Deep Learning for Neurodegenerative Disease Targets

Neurodegenerative disorders, including Alzheimer's and Parkinson's diseases, present hurdles when identifying targets because these diseases have multiple causes and obtain scarce biopsy materials. In this case study, researchers implemented a deep neural network (DNN) trained on single-cell RNA sequencing data, GWAS datasets, and brain-specific interactomes to identify novel protein targets associated with disease progression [8].

Unsupervised learning methods with clustering techniques enabled the model to identify differences between neurons having disease vs. healthy states while indicating proteins with both population-level variations and strong network integration roles. Several receptors associated with microglia and synaptic proteins which the AI system anticipated led to neurodegenerative validation when tested in transgenic mouse models.

This case study illustrates how AI can integrate disparate and complex neurological datasets to unravel the molecular underpinnings of brain disorders, opening avenues for precision-targeted interventions.

AI in Drug Repurposing

Drug repurposing as a method to repurpose existing drugs as new therapeutic applications has become highly popular because it reduces development costs while shortening research timelines and presents lower clinical risks. The development of AI produced powerful tools which extract data-driven hypotheses at high speeds from extensive biomedical information repositories. By using pattern recognition, network modeling, and ML algorithms, AI can uncover hidden associations between drugs, diseases, and molecular targets that would be difficult to detect using conventional methods [9].

Case Study 3: COVID-19 and Rapid AI-Based Repurposing

The worldwide COVID-19 crisis demanded efficient therapeutic solutions at an unprecedented speed. Researchers founded AI-powered platforms to scan thousands of available compounds against SARS-CoV-2. A pioneering study applied deep learning technology to molecular docking predictions for discovering drug-virus binding possibilities.

The AI system integrated data from viral protein structures, known drug-target interaction databases, and host-pathogen interaction networks. The model used during this process found several potential drugs in less than a week with remdesivir and baricitinib among them as well as camostat mesylate. The drugs destined for clinical trials or emergency use authorizations started their path through fast processes. This case showcases the quick response and numerous benefits that AI offers when it uses intelligent drug repositioning to handle worldwide health emergencies [10].

Case Study 4: Rare Diseases and Knowledge Graph Applications

Therapeutic attention neglects rare diseases mainly because markets lack enough patients to warrant investment and commercial incentives do not motivate production. The lack of therapeutic attention for rare diseases gets solved through AI by using knowledge graphs semantic networks to create connections between diseases, genes, drugs and phenotypes.

In this case study, a research team constructed a comprehensive biomedical knowledge graph integrating literature mining, EHRs, genomic annotations, and clinical trial databases. Using GNNs, the model predicted previously unrecognized drug-disease associations in rare genetic disorders like Gaucher disease and Duchenne muscular dystrophy [11].

The AI platform proposed using miglustat and tacrolimus through an analysis based on matching pathways and expression profiles between genes. Testing results obtained through in vitro assays confirmed the earlier discovered relationships. Knowledge graph-based AI provides a mechanism to reveal concealed disease connections which thereby reveals new therapeutic approaches for abandoned diseases.

AI for Hit Identification and Lead Optimization

Early drug discovery depends heavily on hit identification and lead optimization because these two steps identify potential active molecules for biological targets followed by their development into drug candidate substances. The standard practice of HTS and iterative medicinal chemistry takes up plenty of time and costs significant amounts of money in these processes. AI, particularly through generative models and reinforcement learning (RL), offers transformative capabilities to accelerate and enhance these stages by enabling intelligent molecule design, predictive scoring, and multi-objective optimization [12].

Case Study 5: Generative Models for Novel Compound Generation

AI-generated models, including VAEs, GANs, and transformers, gain increasing popularity in the development of new chemical compounds possessing required biologically active and physical chemical properties. A VAE-based framework operated through training on a big collection of bioactive compounds expressed in Simplified Molecular Input Line Entry System (SMILES) format.

By conditioning the generative process on specific molecular features like logP, binding affinity, and toxicity profile, the model was able to produce novel chemical scaffolds predicted to bind with high affinity to oncogenic kinases. The study team synthesized multiple potential active candidates and tested them by performing in vitro experiments which revealed two compounds exhibited below micromolar strength and suitable ADMET attributes. The implementation demonstrates how AI technologies can urgently cut the time required for developing new drugs from conceptualization to production.

Case Study 6: Reinforcement Learning in Lead Optimization

Lead optimization requires fine-tuning of hit compounds to improve potency, selectivity, solubility, and safety. In this case, an RL approach was adopted, where an AI agent learned to make chemical modifications on a lead scaffold to maximize a reward function comprising multiple drug-like properties [13].

The RL model utilized three reward metrics of docking scores alongside synthetic accessibility scores and predicted off-target to search across extensive areas of chemical space through its virtual synthesis process. The model produced new chemical derivatives from a neuroinflammation receptor lead compound which showcased better binding properties while displaying reduced heart toxic effects.

Several of the optimized leads progressed to in vivo pharmacokinetic and efficacy studies, outperforming the parent compound. The case demonstrates that RL

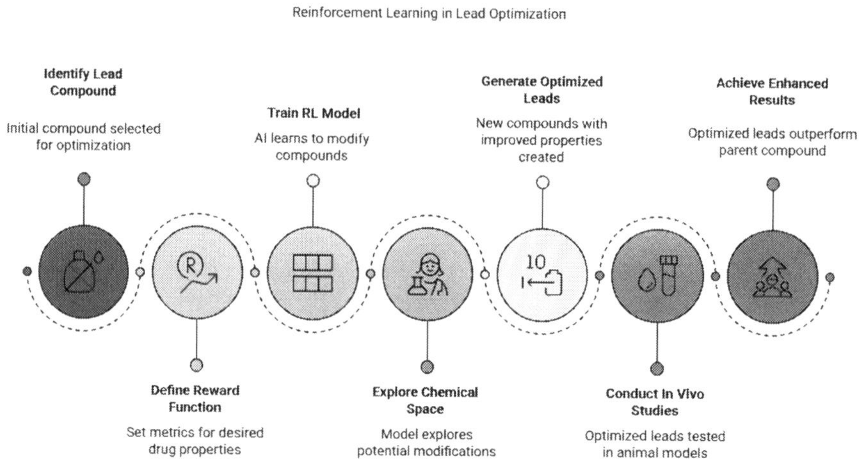

Figure 8.2 Reinforcement Learning in Lead Optimization

together with AI allows computers to perform systematic chemical modification searches, which optimizes lead compounds more effectively (Figure 8.2).

Predictive Toxicology and ADMET Profiling

Traditionally, the ADME and toxicity properties of compounds need to be determined early during drug discovery to prevent costly late stage failures. The traditional ADMET evaluation process requires labor-intensive and time-consuming in vitro and in vivo testing procedures. AI has emerged as a robust tool to predict ADMET and toxicological profiles using in silico models trained on historical data, offering faster, cost-effective, and scalable alternatives [14].

Case Study 7: In Silico ADMET Screening Using AI Pipelines

To evaluate the ADMET properties of the 10,000 virtual compounds, an integrated AI system was built. Doctors used the pipeline that merged random forest and SVM and GBM algorithms to analyze datasets obtained from ChEMBL and Tox21 and DrugBank.

The models evaluated a range of parameters, including oral bioavailability, blood-brain barrier permeability, metabolic stability, and hepatotoxicity. The presynthesis filtering process removed compounds with low ADMET attributes scores which reduced the whole experimental work. The prediction methodology achieved high accuracy during retrospective validation because it matched experimental results correctly more than 85% of the time. This case highlights how AI-powered virtual screening can de-risk early phase discovery and improve the selection of lead candidates [15].

Case Study 8: Predicting Cardiotoxicity Using Convolutional Neural Networks

The primary underlying reason which forces pharmaceutical companies to remove drugs from their markets is toxic effects on heart tissue which frequently stems from hERG channel impairments. This research developed a CNN system which combined electromyographic test results with molecular signature sequences to detect small molecule cardiac toxicity potential.

The CNN model extracted spatial patterns from compound structures and electrophysiological datasets to learn complex relationships indicative of cardiotoxic potential. The model demonstrated superior performance by achieving an AUC of 0.92 for determining cardiotoxic liabilities within a blinded test of new molecules above traditional QSAR models. The explainability feature of the AI model enabled researchers to detect molecular features linked with risk so medicinal chemists could utilize this data for practical actions [16].

AI in Preclinical and Clinical Trial Design

Drug development reaches its most expensive and time-consuming stage during clinical trials while maintaining high rates of candidate drug failure. The combination of predictive modeling and real-time data analysis through AI creates a revolutionary capability which transforms trial planning and operation and analysis processes to deliver smarter decision support. From patient stratification to adaptive trial designs, AI tools are helping pharmaceutical companies accelerate timelines while improving safety and efficacy outcomes.

Case Study 9: Patient Stratification Using AI

The nature of different patients present challenges during clinical trials because it weakens therapeutic effects while making treatment assessment more complicated. Use of AI technology allowed researchers to group metastatic breast cancer patients through a combination of genomic data together with clinical information as well as imaging results. A multi-modal neural network was trained on historical trial datasets to identify patient subpopulations most likely to respond to a novel immunotherapy [17].

The model processed predicted and classified patients into distinct response groups by running supervised classification with unsupervised clustering. The systematic patient grouping through stratification resulted in better trial success rates with higher response rates of 30% and smaller trial populations by 20%. The trial also benefited from faster enrollment and improved regulatory engagement due to its precision-based design. This case emphasizes the role of AI in personalizing trial enrollment, improving both efficiency and success rates.

Case Study 10: Adaptive Trial Design Optimization with Machine Learning

Adaptive trials provide mutable protocol modifications which depend on provisional data in order to enhance standard ethical practices and trial flexibility. The authors implemented ML algorithms to create simulated trials for assessing different situations involving a novel anti-inflammatory drug. The system evaluated outcomes, such as dosage adjustments, cohort expansions, and endpoint refinements using RL techniques [18].

Bayesian optimization ran as a framework above the simulation to give dynamic adjustment recommendations that maintained statistical integrity. This AI-powered design executed during Phase II testing minimized clinical investigations by six months while achieving an improvement of 15% regarding power for identifying significant differences between groups.

This case underscores how AI can make clinical trials more dynamic, responsive, and data-driven, significantly increasing the probability of regulatory approval and market success.

Integration of AI with Omics and Systems Biology

Medical sciences have advanced remarkably with AI joining forces with omics technologies, such as genomics transcriptomics proteomics and metabolomics to analyze biological systems more effectively. AI-powered systems biology techniques generate mathematical frameworks to depict complete biological pathways which deliver an integrated knowledge about medical conditions and drug reactions. This integration is particularly powerful in identifying biomarkers, predicting drug efficacy, and designing combination therapies based on mechanistic insights [19].

Case Study 11: Multi-Omics Fusion for Biomarker Discovery

ML algorithms combined three types of omic datasets (transcriptomics, proteomics, and metabolomics) extracted from pancreatic cancer patients at its initial stages. During analysis, the DL framework processed high-dimensional data to find delicate disease development indicators.

Using autoencoders and attention-based neural networks, the model was able to identify a panel of predictive biomarkers with high sensitivity and specificity. The validated markers are currently developed for use as part of a diagnostic assay. The research method achieved better results than conventional single-omics tests because AI demonstrated its ability to find meaningful biological signals in highly complex datasets [20].

This case illustrates the transformative potential of AI in precision medicine, offering a path toward early detection and individualized treatment strategies.

Case Study 12: AI in Network Pharmacology for Drug Combination Strategies

The development of drugs through system biology benefits heavily from AI which helps discover potent drug mixes. The evaluation of drug interactions inside non-small cell lung cancer signaling pathways was conducted through experiments that linked GNNs and network pharmacology models.

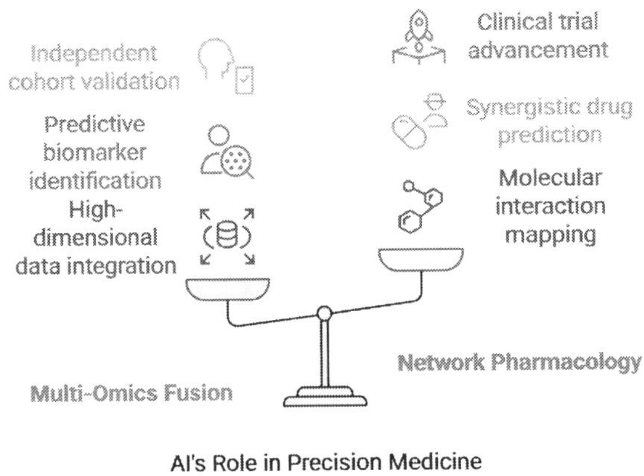

Figure 8.3 AI's Role in Precision Medicine

The model mapped molecular interactions and integrated clinical response data to identify optimal drug pairs that could jointly modulate critical nodes in the disease network. RL algorithms iteratively improved prediction accuracy based on in vitro validation feedback [21].

Multiple new drug pairings from the approach proceeded into clinical trials during their early phase. This case demonstrates that systems biology combined with AI leads to logical combination therapy design specially beneficial for treating difficult complex diseases (Figure 8.3).

Industry Use Cases and Success Stories

Various biotech and pharmaceutical businesses are implementing AI-driven platforms in their R&D pipelines since drug discovery applications of AI have witnessed a rapid commercial expansion. This explores how cutting-edge companies are leveraging AI for real-world breakthroughs, highlighting two prominent case studies that demonstrate innovation, scalability, and clinical relevance [22].

Case Study 13: BenevolentAI's Approach to Automated Hypothesis Generation

BenevolentAI is a frontrunner in AI-driven hypothesis generation, utilizing DL and NLP to mine vast biomedical datasets, including literature, clinical trial data, and molecular databases. Through its AI platform, the company builds dynamic knowledge graphs that represented disease mechanisms as well as biological pathways and compound interactions.

BenevolentAI employed its AI system to quickly find baricitinib as a potential countermeasure for virus-induced cytokine storm because of the COVID-19 pandemic. The AI model linked separated data points across virologic, immunologic, and pharmacologic fields to generate the new treatment approach that medical institutions confirmed in clinical practice and added to official healthcare protocols.

This success illustrates how AI can accelerate hypothesis formation, drastically reduce discovery timelines, and guide strategic decision-making in real-world settings [23].

Case Study 14: Atomwise's Structure-Based Drug Screening Platform

Atomwise made a groundbreaking discovery through its development of CNNs for the purposes of virtual screening and molecular docking. The AtomNet® platform from Atomwise predicts binding affinity as well as molecular interactions by processing 3D structural data of protein-ligand complexes.

One of Atomwise's most notable successes involved identifying potential inhibitors for Ebola virus proteins in a matter of days an effort that would have traditionally taken months. The platform has also been used in collaboration with more than 750 partners, including academic labs, biotech firms, and pharmaceutical companies, across a wide range of therapeutic areas.

Drugs identified through Atomwise operations perform incredible target structure searches that handle massive compound numbers with precision, thus making the hit identification process much quicker and effective. The predictive power of AtomNet along with its ability to scale up is revolutionizing drug discovery during its early development stages by speeding up the entire process [24].

Regulatory and Ethical Considerations

The growing presence of AI technologies within drug discovery pipelines requires concentrated efforts from regulatory agencies and ethical guidelines for proper oversight. This examines the critical dimensions of data transparency, model explainability, and regulatory frameworks necessary to ensure responsible and trustworthy AI adoption in pharmaceutical research.

Data Transparency and Model Interpretability

AI models that work in drug discovery require extensive datasets comprising omics information and clinical trial statistics as well as EHR recordings. Transparency in data requires full documentation of training and validation databases which should be easily tracked with clear identification of potential influences that could impact generalization or outcome results. The ability to interpret the models proves critical for winning regulatory institution approval as well as trust from both researchers and medical clinicians. Black-box models that yield predictions without offering insight into how decisions are made are particularly problematic in a highly regulated domain like healthcare [25].

The FDA and EMA have launched current initiatives to encourage researchers to deploy interpretable AI systems because AI decision outputs require transparency. AI workflows adopt the SHAP and LIME techniques to improve the explainability of decision systems for enhancing both translation and accountability (Table 8.3).

Table 8.3 Regulatory and Ethical Factors in AI

Aspect	*Challenge*	*AI Solution*	*Regulatory Outlook*
Transparency	Black-box models	Explainable AI (XAI)	Ongoing evaluation
Data Bias	Limited demographic data	Balanced datasets	Draft FDA guidance emerging
Accountability	Model misjudgment	Human-in-loop validation	Required under GxP

AI Explainability in Decision-Making

Reliable incorporation of AI technology into decision-making systems requires explainable reasoning to satisfy technical and non-technical stakeholders who evaluate drug candidate selection and patient stratification processes. The requirement to make AI systems explainable constitutes a vital ethical requirement as well as a functional prerequisite. The lack of understanding regarding predictions made by the model results in improper clinical decisions as well as patient mistrust and actual harm.

In response, regulatory bodies are beginning to require "algorithmic audit trails" records that show how AI decisions were derived. Such requirements ensure transparency and support post hoc analyses if adverse outcomes occur. The necessity of explainability becomes crucial in adaptive trial design and AI diagnosis tools since it enables proper compliance along with patient consent processes and autonomy amounts [26].

Regulatory Acceptance Frameworks

Current regulatory agencies face ongoing challenges to develop proper acceptance guidelines for AI programs because of fast-paced technological progress. The FDA implements the "Action Plan for Artificial Intelligence/Machine Learning-Based Software as a Medical Device" to provide pre-market and post-market oversight procedures. Frameworks resembling these ones are being implemented throughout Europe as well as Japan and India.

Key components of regulatory evaluation include:

- Data integrity and traceability
- Model performance across populations
- Risk management strategies
- Continuous learning system safeguards

A practice known as Good Machine Learning Practice (GMLP) seeks to unite AI development with established good manufacturing practices (GMP) in the pharmaceutical sector. The planned collaboration between AI tools and traditional methods guarantees their precise functionality as well as their safety and their ability to give reliable results after deployment [27].

Challenges and Future Perspectives

The path of drug discovery transformation through AI requires both an investigation of integration obstacles and forecasts about upcoming changes. This discusses present shortcomings of AI systems and human-machine intelligence dynamics while examining future directions in medicine utilization of AI for individualized care.

Limitations in Data Quality and Algorithmic Bias

One of the primary obstacles in AI-driven drug discovery is the quality, diversity, and representativeness of data. Biomedical datasets often suffer from incompleteness, inconsistency, and noise. The same data obtained from public domains shows insufficient annotation details and maintains biased elements which become more prominent within particular ethnic groups and healthcare settings. RLS systems transfer erroneous information from their training data which typically results in inaccurate predictions and unpropitious healthcare results [28].

Moreover, imbalanced datasets where positive outcomes are overrepresented can mislead algorithms and reduce the reliability of drug efficacy or toxicity predictions. The prevention of algorithmic biases requires both improved data cleansing processes and new detection tools for detecting algorithmic biases along with stronger data sharing protocols.

Integration with Human Intelligence and Automation

Reliable incorporation of AI technology into decision-making systems requires explainable reasoning to satisfy technical and non-technical stakeholders who evaluate drug candidate selection and patient stratification processes. The requirement to make AI systems explainable constitutes a vital ethical requirement as well as a functional prerequisite. The lack of understanding regarding predictions made by the model results in improper clinical decisions as well as patient mistrust and actual harm.

Simultaneously, automation powered by AI from HTS to digital lab assistants is set to revolutionize drug pipelines. The necessity of explainability becomes crucial in adaptive trial design and AI diagnosis tools since it enables proper compliance along with patient consent processes and autonomy amounts [29].

Future Directions: AI in Personalized and Precision Medicine

The swift technological progress has not kept pace with regulatory bodies which are developing their acceptance standards for AI solutions. The FDA implements the "Action Plan for Artificial Intelligence/Machine Learning-Based Software as a Medical Device" to provide pre-market and post-market oversight procedures. Frameworks resembling these ones are being implemented throughout Europe as well as Japan and India.

AI models will play a vital role in predictive diagnostics, dynamic treatment planning, and real-time monitoring of therapeutic efficacy. With the convergence of AI, CRISPR, and nanotechnology, we can envision a future where drugs are not just discovered but intelligently designed and adapted in real time for each patient [30].

Conclusion

The ongoing reshaping of drug discovery by AI requires researchers to analyze current barriers for complete implementation along with predictions about upcoming developments. The research examines present AI implementation barriers together with human-computer intelligence dynamics and future AI-driven developments in managing personalized medical care.

Summarizing Insights from the Case Studies

The same data obtained from public domains shows insufficient annotation details and maintains biased elements which become more prominent within particular ethnic groups and healthcare settings. RLS systems transfer erroneous information from their training data which typically results in inaccurate predictions and unpropitious healthcare results. AI has demonstrated remarkable capability in:

- Identifying novel and previously undruggable targets (e.g., kinases and neurological biomarkers),
- Repurposing existing drugs with new therapeutic potential, especially during urgent health crises like COVID-19,
- Designing novel chemical entities through GANs and RL strategies,
- Enhancing preclinical and clinical trial efficiencies through improved patient stratification and adaptive design,
- Predicting safety profiles and pharmacokinetic parameters with greater accuracy using in silico methods.

These successes have significantly accelerated the pace of drug discovery, improved the precision of therapeutic interventions, and reduced costs and attrition rates within pharmaceutical pipelines [31].

The Evolving Paradigm of AI-Powered Drug Discovery

AI drug discovery continues to advance because of better computational capabilities along with expanding quality dataset availability and rising acceptance of digital technologies in regulatory and clinical frameworks. Various medical professionals working together prove indispensable for converting AI-derived knowledge into functional healthcare solutions.

Looking ahead, AI will not merely assist in drug development it will co-create and personalize therapies in a truly patient-centric model. The growing capability of AI systems to be explained and integrated with regulatory structures will boost healthcare trust in these systems as well as their useful application [32].

This provides both a portfolio of significant case research and evidence that AI drives transformative breakthroughs in developing new drugs. So far just the start of what will turn out to be transformational advancements resulting from interweaving algorithms with biology and human intuition.

References

1. DiMasi, J. A., Grabowski, H. G., & Hansen, R. W. (2016). Innovation in the pharmaceutical industry: New estimates of R&D costs. *Journal of Health Economics*, *47*, 20–33.
2. Wouters, O. J., McKee, M., & Luyten, J. (2020). Estimated research and development investment needed to bring a new medicine to market, 2009–2018. *JAMA*, *323*(9), 844–853.
3. Aminabee, S. K., Prabhakar, M. C., Prasad, R. G. S. V., & Lakshmana Rao, A. (2011). Screening the pharmacological activity of cerium oxide nanoparticles in-vitro. *Biomedical and Pharmacology Journal*, *4*(2), 287–289.
4. Lavecchia, A., & Di Giovanni, C. (2013). Virtual screening strategies in drug discovery: A critical review. *Current Medicinal Chemistry*, *20*(23), 2839–2860.
5. Aminabee, S. K., Lakshmana Rao, A., Sowmya, K., Nymisha, D., Kusuma Naga Lakshmi, K., Manikanta, K. V. N. S., & Praveen Kumar, P. (2019). Evaluation of analgesic activity of *Ficus palmata*. *Iranian Journal of Pharmaceutical Sciences*, *15*(3), 47–60.
6. Wang, J., Wolf, R. M., Caldwell, J. W., Kollman, P. A., & Case, D. A. (2004). Development and testing of a general AMBER force field. *Journal of Computational Chemistry*, *25*(9), 1157–1174.
7. Vanommeslaeghe, K., et al. (2010). CHARMM general force field: A force field for drug-like molecules compatible with the CHARMM all-atom additive biological force fields. *Journal of Computational Chemistry*, *31*(4), 671–690.
8. Aminabee, S. K., Lakshmana Rao, A., & Chinna Eswaraiah, M. (2020). In-vivo antioxidant activity of different fractions of *Indigofera barberi* against paracetamol-induced toxicity in rats. *Turkish Journal of Pharmaceutical Sciences*, *17*(2), 136–140.
9. Yang, S. Y. (2010). Pharmacophore modeling and applications in drug discovery: Challenges and recent advances. *Drug Discovery Today*, *15*(11–12), 444–450.
10. Prasanth, D. S. N. B. K., Aminabee, S. K., Lakshmana Rao, A., Teja, N., Bhargavi, K., Monika, C., Pujitha, B., Sandhya, T., Lalitha, A., & Siva Prasad, P. (2020). Anthelmintic activity of *Mansoa alliacea* against *Pheretima posthuma*: In-vitro and in-silico approach. *Thai Journal of Pharmaceutical Sciences*, *4*(3), 186–196.
11. Muegge, I., & Mukherjee, P. (2016). An overview of molecular fingerprint similarity search in virtual screening. *Expert Opinion on Drug Discovery*, *11*(2), 137–148.
12. Lavecchia, A. (2015). Machine-learning approaches in drug discovery: Methods and applications. *Drug Discovery Today*, *20*(3), 318–331.
13. Prasanth, D. S. N. B. K., Aminabee, S. K., Lakshmana Rao, A., Guntupalli, C., Reddy, A. R., Kulandaivelu, U., Rao, S. N. K., & Rajeshwari, P. (2021). Inhibitory effects of *Mansoa alliacea* in Freund's adjuvant arthritis on inflammatory markers and its confirmation by in-silico strategy. *Thai Journal of Pharmaceutical Sciences*, *45*(6), 532–544.
14. Aliper, A., Plis, S., Artemov, A., Ulloa, A., Mamoshina, P., & Zhavoronkov, A. (2016). Deep learning applications for predicting pharmacological properties of drugs and drug repurposing using transcriptomic data. *Molecular Pharmaceutics*, *13*(7), 2524–2530.
15. Aminabee, S. K., Santhi Krupa, D., Hanumanth Rao, K., Sirisha, V., Anitha Kumari, V., Nagasen, D., Sujiya, B., & Leelavati, T. S. (2023). Pharmacoeconomic analysis of biologic vs. biosimilar therapies in rheumatoid arthritis. *International Journal of Chemical and Biochemical Sciences*, *24*(4), 395–400.

16. Romanelli, V., Cerchia, C., & Lavecchia, A. (2024). Unlocking the potential of generative artificial intelligence in drug discovery. In *Applications of Generative AI* (pp. 37–63).
17. Cerchia, C., & Lavecchia, A. (2023). New avenues in artificial-intelligence-assisted drug discovery. *Drug Discovery Today*, *28*, 103516.
18. Karras, T., Laine, S., Aittala, M., Hellsten, J., Lehtinen, J., & Aila, T. (2020). Analyzing and improving the image quality of StyleGAN. In *2020 IEEE/CVF Conference on Computer Vision and Pattern Recognition (CVPR)* (pp. 8107–8116). IEEE.
19. Leelavati, T. S., Madhavi, S., Kamal, G., Raju, P. V. M., Susmitha, K., Vinod, M., & Aminabee, S. K. (2023). Revolutionizing healthcare delivery: Telemedicine's influence on access and patient satisfaction. *International Journal of Chemical and Biochemical Sciences*, *24*(5), 106–115.
20. Zhavoronkov, A., et al. (2019). Deep learning enables rapid identification of potent DDR1 kinase inhibitors. *Nature Biotechnology*, *37*(9), 1038–1040.
21. Aminabee, S. K., Devi Mallika, K., & Lakshmana Rao, A. (2023). Natural resources in management and treatment of diseases: A review. *Pharma Times*, *55*(11), 7–10.
22. David, L., Thakkar, A., Mercado, R., & Engkvist, O. (2020). Molecular representations in AI-driven drug discovery: A review and practical guide. *Journal of Cheminformatics*, *12*, 56.
23. Loeffler, H. H., He, J., Tibo, A., Janet, J. P., Voronov, A., Mervin, L. H., & Engvist, O. (2024). Reinvent 4: Modern AI-driven generative molecule design. *Journal of Cheminformatics*, *16*, 20.
24. O'Boyle, N., & Dalke, A. (2018). DeepSMILES: An adaptation of SMILES for use in machine-learning of chemical structures. *ChemRxiv*.
25. Aminabee, S. K., & Lakshmana Rao, A. (2024). Computational identification of selected bioactive compounds from *Cedrus deodara* as inhibitors against SARS-CoV-2 main protease: A pharmacoinformatics study. *Indian Drugs*, *61*(2), 78–91.
26. Yuan, Z., & Briscoe, T. (2016). Grammatical error correction using neural machine translation. In *Proceedings of the 2016 Conference of the North American Chapter of the Association for Computational Linguistics: Human Language Technologies* (pp. 380–386).
27. Zheng, S., Rao, J., Zhang, Z., Xu, J., & Yang, Y. (2019). Predicting retrosynthetic reactions using self-corrected transformer neural networks. *Journal of Chemical Information and Modeling*, *60*(1), 47–55.
28. Ravi Shankar, K., Aminabee, S. K., Ramana, G., Chenchu Lakshmi, K. N. V., & Indusree, G. (2024). Formulation and evaluation of propranolol hydrochloride floating tablets by 32 factorial design. *International Journal of Drug Delivery Technology*, *14*(4), 2060–2067.
29. Sun, Z., Zhu, Q., Mou, L., Xiong, Y., Li, G., & Zhang, L. (2018). A grammar-based structural CNN decoder for code generation. In AAAI Conference on Artificial Intelligence.
30. Hadjeres, G., & Nielsen, F. (2020). Anticipation-RNN: Enforcing unary constraints in sequence generation, with application to interactive music generation. *Neural Computing and Applications*, *32*, 995–1005.
31. Hochreiter, S., & Schmidhuber, J. (1997). Long short-term memory. *Neural Computation*, *9*(8), 1735–1780.
32. Cho, K., van Merrienboer, B., Gulcehre, C., Bahdanau, D., Bougares, F., Schwenk, H., & Bengio, Y. (2014). Learning phrase representations using RNN encoder-decoder for statistical machine translation. *arXiv*.

9 Future Trends in AI-Powered Drug Discovery

Introduction

Evolution of Drug Discovery and the Emergence of AI

The discovery methods behind pharmaceutical development have experienced a major shift throughout the last hundred years that transformed accidental discoveries into focused target-based strategies. Drug discovery followed a lengthy delay-and-error approach until scientific progress through organic chemistry and pharmacology provided better support yet the process continued to cause extensive delays and many abandoned projects. The emergence of Artificial Intelligence (AI) has marked a paradigm shift in this field. AI technologies particularly machine learning (ML) and deep learning (DL) offer the ability to process and learn from vast, complex datasets, identifying patterns and relationships that are often invisible to traditional analytical methods. Drugs discovery features a major change at different points along the research process because these technologies revolutionize target identification as well as compound screening and toxicity prediction and clinical trial optimization [1].

Role of Big Data and Multi-Omics in Enabling AI Applications

Drug discovery capitalizes on the large explosion of biomedical data and becomes the perfect environment for AI system integration. Next-generation sequencing (NGS) mass spectrometry and high-content screening systems produce enormous datasets that span genomics transcriptomics proteomics metabolomics and epigenomics studies which researchers refer to as multi-omics data. These datasets, when effectively integrated and analyzed, provide a comprehensive view of biological systems at the molecular level. AI models, particularly those based on neural networks and natural language processing (NLP), can digest and interpret this data to uncover novel disease mechanisms, identify druggable targets, and predict therapeutic responses. AI benefits from the increasing quantity of clinical data derived from electronic health records (EHRs) coupled with real-world evidence and wearable devices to develop exact drugs that apply to individual patient needs (Figure 9.1).

DOI: 10.4324/9781003616177-9

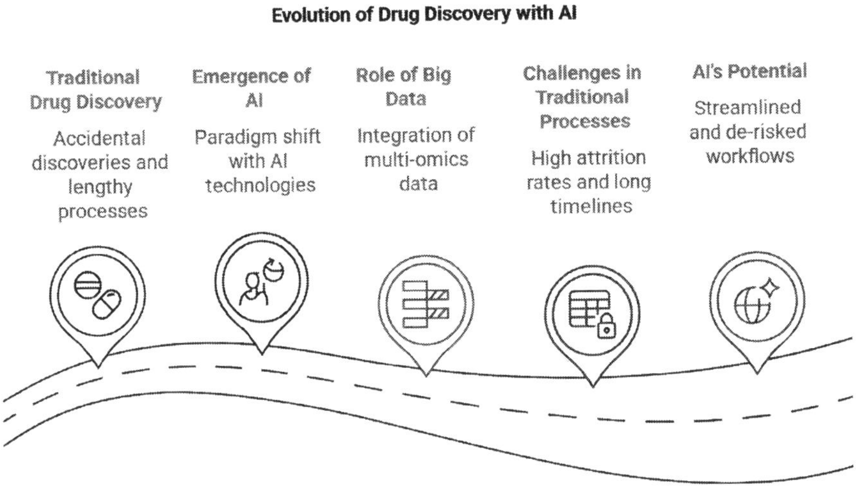

Figure 9.1 Evolution of Drug Discovery with AI

Challenges in Traditional Drug Discovery Pipelines

The continuous development of technology has not solved fundamental problems affecting traditional drug discovery processes. The development timeline between target identification and market approval spans over 12 years along with expenditure reaching billions of dollars. One of the key bottlenecks is the high attrition rate of candidate molecules, often due to unforeseen toxicity, lack of efficacy, or poor pharmacokinetic properties that only become apparent in late stage clinical trials. Human diseases particularly those occurring as polygenic and multifactorial disorders become difficult to model precisely through traditional methods. The constrained data segregation together with disciplinary division and reductionist operational framework functions as barriers for innovation [2]. Several drug discovery process barriers should become less challenging because AI can unite extensive data sources and find hidden patterns and create new hypotheses at massive proportions. This potential capability suggests better streamlined de risked medicine development workflows.

The Current Landscape of AI in Drug Discovery

Overview of AI Tools (ML, DL, NLP, Reinforcement Learning)

AI in drug discovery leverages a spectrum of computational tools, each with distinct capabilities. Healthcare developers implement ML techniques as the fundamental component of AI drug development to discover hidden patterns in biomedical data which yields forecasts about drug activities and adverse effects and binding site behaviors. DL, a subset of ML, employs multi-layered neural networks capable of modeling intricate, non-linear relationships in large datasets, making it especially useful for image analysis, protein folding prediction, and de novo molecule design. NLP technology allows machines to extract valuable information from unorganized text which includes scientific literature and clinical trial reports, thus enabling scientists to generate hypotheses and identify their targets [3]. The drug design optimization process benefits from using Reinforcement Learning (RL) which enables decision-making through experimental trials to generate pharmaceutically suitable molecules.

Integration with Cheminformatics and Bioinformatics

AI applications in drug discovery require a strong connection with cheminformatics and bioinformatics to achieve successful implementation. The application of computational analysis tools through cheminformatics supports chemical data management and visualizes data to execute methods, such as virtual screening and molecular docking and quantitative structure-activity relationship (QSAR) modeling tasks. AI enhances these tasks by improving prediction accuracy and reducing the time required for lead optimization. Similarly, bioinformatics focuses on interpreting biological data particularly from genomic, transcriptomic, and proteomic sources. ML tools serve three vital functions: they reveal new paths of disease progression and they help predict genetic-disease linkages between sequences while tracking suitable diagnostic or therapeutic biomarkers [4]. Through their combined use, AI tools enhance a comprehensive research method that merges chemical database information with biological operation data to help develop drugs while maintaining high precision.

Major Achievements and Case Studies (e.g., AlphaFold, Exscientia, and BenevolentAI)

Several landmark achievements have underscored the potential of AI in transforming drug discovery. AlphaFold from DeepMind stands as a transformative discovery in protein structure prediction by delivering forecasts that equal live experimental definitiveness concerning protein three-dimensional shapes. This breakthrough has unlocked new possibilities in understanding disease mechanisms and designing structure-based therapeutics. Companies like Exscientia and BenevolentAI have further demonstrated the power of AI in real-world drug development. Exscientia implements AI to produce molecules with perfect pharmacokinetic and pharmacodynamic features which cuts the pharmaceutical development process down [5]. One of its AI-researched drugs completed its way to clinical trials at an unprecedented pace. The ML systems at BenevolentAI combined with their knowledge graphs help discover new pharmaceutical targets alongside their role in finding possible COVID-19 treatments. These case studies exemplify how AI is no longer a theoretical tool but a practical, impactful component of modern pharmaceutical research (Table 9.1).

Table 9.1 Major Achievements and Case Studies in AI Drug Discovery

Platform/Study	*AI Tool Used*	*Application*	*Key Achievement*
AlphaFold	Deep Learning	Protein structure prediction	Successfully predicted 3D structures of proteins with high accuracy.
Exscientia	Deep Learning, Reinforcement Learning	Lead compound design and optimization	Developed AI-designed drug candidate (EXS-21546) entering clinical trials.
BenevolentAI	Machine Learning, NLP	Drug discovery, biomarker identification	Identified a potential treatment for autoimmune diseases.
Insilico Medicine	Deep Learning, Generative Models	Drug discovery and aging research	AI discovered a novel drug for fibrosis treatment, currently in clinical trials.

AI in Target Identification and Validation

Mining Genomics, Proteomics, and Transcriptomics Data

Drug discovery starts with precisely validating and confirming therapeutic targets which represent the initial fundamental step. The analytical phase benefits from AI which efficiently analyzes complex omics datasets that consist of genomics and proteomics and transcriptomics forms. The DNA-based disease association data from genomics and the identification of pathological state-dependent gene expression through transcriptomics help scientists develop disease-understanding. Proteomics focuses on the protein expression and interaction landscape, offering clues about functional and structural roles in disease progression [6]. Traditional methods often struggle with the volume and complexity of such datasets. AI effectively detects obscure yet crucial relationships between data points, which leads to elevated target identification accuracy and processes.

AI-Based Identification of Novel Disease Pathways and Biomarkers

The identification of new disease mechanisms benefits vastly from AI methods which use ML and DL as their core components. AI models which analyze multiple types of biological data enable forecasting between disease phenotype responses and certain genes or proteins allowing scientists to detect key points in disease pathways. These insights lead to the discovery of novel pathways that may not be evident through conventional analysis. AI systems efficiently generate reliable biomarkers which function as biological signs that indicate disease status and its evolution and treatment reaction. Biomarkers serve fundamental functions to improve diagnostic assessment and determine prognosis outcomes while they help define patient groups in clinical experiments [7]. AI speeds up biomarker research while making newly discovered biomarkers more precise through extensive data-based testing.

Use of Graph Neural Networks (GNNs) and Knowledge Graphs

Target identification advances through implementation of Graph Neural Networks (GNNs) together with knowledge graphs. The complex non-linear nature of biological system relationships makes GNNs the perfect tool for modeling such biological systems. GNNs learn from both the attributes of biological entities and the structure of their interactions, enabling more nuanced predictions about potential drug targets. Knowledge graphs, however, compile structured biomedical knowledge from diverse sources literature, databases, and clinical data into interconnected nodes and edges. These algorithms explore such interactive networks to identify unnoticed connections and determine critical objectives and produce explanatory descriptions about disease characteristics [8]. GNNs combined with knowledge graphs supply AI-driven drug discovery with an advanced tool set that optimizes the reliability and innovation process for identifying therapeutic targets (Figure 9.2).

AI in Lead Compound Identification and Optimization

Deep Generative Models (VAEs, GANs) for De Novo Molecule Design

Among the leading AI-based approaches for de novo drug designing stand deep generative models which include Variational Autoencoders (VAEs) and Generative Adversarial Networks (GANs). The models process massive chemical datasets to produce new molecular structures which follow desired drug-related characteristics. The encoding process of molecules into latent space combined with variant decoding operates through controlled chemical space exploration. GANs, comprising a generator and discriminator network in a competitive setup, can create highly realistic and structurally valid compounds [9]. The implementation of AI methods

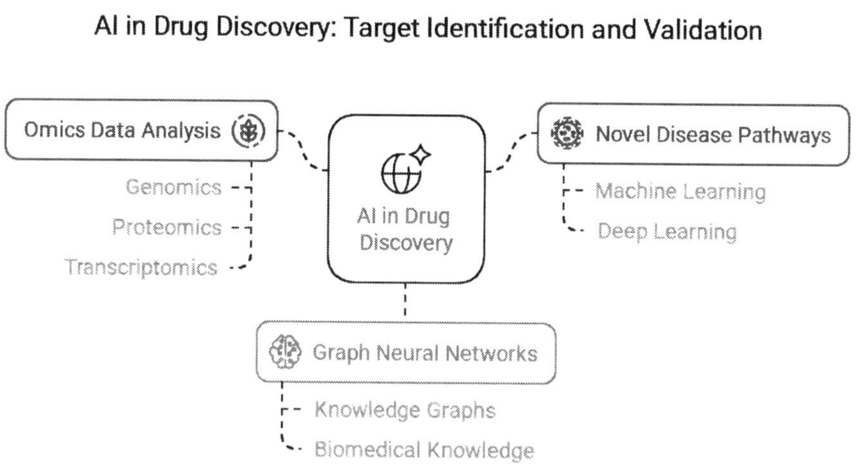

Figure 9.2 Redefining Drug Discovery with AI

decreases time and resource requirements to evaluate chemical space so researchers can identify innovative lead compounds which fulfill both drug-likeness attributes and indicators of synthetic feasibility.

Transfer Learning and Multitask Learning in QSAR Modeling

QSAR modeling gains substantial benefits through the implementation of transfer learning and multitask learning AI methods. Transfer learning enables chemical models from broad generic datasets to adapt their functionality for dealing with rare target properties through fine-tuning even with minimal data availability. This approach improves prediction accuracy and model generalizability. Multitask learning, however, enables simultaneous prediction of multiple biological endpoints or molecular properties, leveraging shared patterns among related tasks [10]. The approach cuts down the need for large labeled datasets per target therefore enabling improved lead determination efficiency within drug discovery development pipelines.

Virtual Screening Using Convolutional Neural Networks (CNNs) and 3D Structure Prediction

The process of lead identification through virtual screening obtains major improvements when utilizing convolutional neural networks (CNNs) together with AI-powered 3D structure prediction methods. The image recognition technique adapted from CNNs applies patterns to either molecular graphs or 3D molecular visuals to estimate binding affinities and biological activity outcomes. These models excel in feature extraction and spatial pattern recognition, improving the accuracy and speed of screening large compound libraries. Coupled with 3D structure prediction techniques, such as those inspired by AlphaFold, AI can model the precise geometry of protein-ligand interactions, thereby refining the selection of lead candidates. The combination of structural bioinformatics with ML technologies provides faster hit-to-lead transition along with improved drug candidates for future stages of drug development [11].

AI for ADMET Prediction

Predictive Modeling for Absorption, Distribution, Metabolism, Excretion, and Toxicity

AI creates revolutionary advancements in the prediction of ADMET profiles for pharmacokinetic and toxicity profiles that represent essential drug safety criteria. ML models, trained on historical pharmacological data, can forecast ADMET properties early in the drug development process, helping to eliminate unsuitable compounds before costly in vitro and in vivo testing. The prediction of solubility together with permeability and plasma protein binding and metabolic stability and hepatotoxicity and cardiotoxicity can be done through the use of random forests

Table 9.2 AI Technologies in ADMET Prediction

Property	*AI Approach*	*Role of AI*	*Challenges*
Absorption	Machine Learning, Deep Learning	Predicting drug absorption based on molecular structure	Difficulty in accurately modeling human physiology.
Distribution	QSAR Modeling, Deep Learning	Modeling drug distribution in different body tissues	Need for better training data across diverse populations.
Metabolism	Machine Learning, Reinforcement Learning	Identifying metabolic pathways and interactions	Incomplete and noisy experimental data.
Excretion	AI-based modeling, Transfer Learning	Predicting excretion profiles based on compound properties	Variability in individual metabolic rates.
Toxicity	Deep Learning, Generative Models	Toxicity prediction based on chemical structures	Lack of high-quality data for training models.

and support vector machines and neural networks algorithms [12]. These predictions significantly enhance decision-making and resource allocation during preclinical evaluation (Table 9.2).

Integration with In Silico PK/PD Modeling

AI-driven ADMET prediction collaborates with in silico pharmacokinetic/pharmacodynamic models for body-based drug candidate dynamic behavior simulation. The use of mechanistic PK/PD models connected to AI-based forecasts enables researchers to design simulations of drug concentration-time profiles in addition to therapeutic windows and dose-response relationships. This integration allows for virtual trials and personalized medicine strategies, reducing the reliance on animal models and expediting clinical translation [13]. Using these technologies together provides researchers with a strong method for devising optimal dose schedules and foreseeing how preclinical findings translate to human results.

Challenges in Dataset Curation and Model Generalizability

The progress made in this field encounters substantial ongoing difficulties when working with available datasets and model applicability to different conditions. The inconsistency together with unbalanced data distribution and nonstandardized assay methods affect the quality of ADMET datasets. Such issues in the data cause biases which diminish both the robustness and reproducibility of AI models. Moreover, the generalizability of models across different chemical spaces, species, or biological systems remains a major hurdle. Steps must contain extensive data cleaning and harmonization protocols together with domain-specific knowledge for making models more interpretable and trustworthy [14]. Inspectable ADMET data sources of high quality need development together with assessment systems to maximize AI utilization across this field.

Reinforcement Learning and Active Learning in Drug Design

Reinforcement Learning Algorithms for Multi-Objective Optimization

Drug design applies RL as one of its most effective AI methods to explore broad chemical domains while respecting multiple design parameters. Within this domain RL agents acquire training to develop or transform molecular structures that fulfill various drug-like requirements which include potency and selectivity and solubility and safety standards. Unlike traditional ML models that rely on static datasets, RL dynamically explores and exploits chemical space by receiving feedback in the form of reward signals based on the desired properties [15]. The method allows researchers to achieve balance in therapeutic compound discovery by finding solutions that benefit their efficacy and their pharmacokinetic performance as well as toxicity factors. Modern RL frameworks deploying both policy gradient approaches and actor-critic frameworks get incorporated into de novo molecular generation platforms to optimize the lead discovery process.

Active Learning to Reduce Experimental Burden

Not only does active learning work alongside RL to resolve the main drug discovery challenge which is experimental data generation costs and time duration but it also provides solutions. Active learning frameworks allow models to decide which compounds provide the best experimental value for validating outcomes while minimizing laboratory expenses. This selective sampling strategy allows researchers to focus experimental efforts on compounds that are expected to provide the most value in refining predictive models [16]. Active learning provides speed to the discovery paradigm while enabling the creation of precise models despite scarce information particularly in fields with minimal research or treatment of rare diseases.

Real-Time Feedback Loops and Adaptive Synthesis Planning

Drug design benefits from real-time feedback loops through the joint application of RL and active learning techniques which enable computational predictions to direct experimental decisions as well as vice versa. A feedback loop operational system enhances drug discovery workflows by enabling quick modifications that stem from experimental data. Additionally, these AI techniques are increasingly being used in adaptive synthesis planning, where the system not only designs novel molecules but also proposes feasible synthetic routes based on available reagents and reaction databases [17]. The end-to-end molecular generation to synthesis planning system shortens development periods and enables practical AI candidate application within pharmaceutical industry operating environments.

Quantum Computing and AI Synergies

Quantum-Enhanced Machine Learning for High-Dimensional Chemical Space

The drug discovery process can transform through quantum computing because it allows scientists to handle greater amounts of chemical data with exceptional processing capabilities. The programs in traditional ML encounter difficulties because of both the vast number of molecular descriptors and structural features that exist in drug-like compounds. Quantum-enhanced machine learning (QML) algorithms, such as quantum support vector machines or quantum kernel methods, can operate in exponentially larger Hilbert spaces, allowing for improved pattern recognition in molecular data [18]. The proposed methods demonstrate promising results when standard computational models experience limitations due to dimensionality so they can speed up and enhance the prediction of molecular properties and binding characteristics.

Hybrid Quantum-Classical Models in Molecular Simulation

Quantum computing combines effectively with AI to enhance molecular simulation processes through hybrid quantum-classical simulation mechanisms. Quantum processors work together with these models to execute simulation tasks for molecular electronic structures and reaction pathways because these operations take too much processing time for conventional computers but they use standard algorithms for optimization along with model assessment. Such integration allows for more precise quantum mechanical modeling of molecular interactions, which is critical in the early stages of drug discovery, such as docking, conformational analysis, and electronic property prediction [19]. Research labs and companies currently explore how quantum variational eigensolvers and quantum Monte Carlo methods can improve pipeline simulation when integrated into AI frameworks for accelerating compound screening.

Future Possibilities and Current Limitations

The attractive theoretical benefits quantum computing and AI could offer together fail to overcome the current operational barriers. Quantum hardware remains at a stage of early development because of challenges involving qubit decoherence together with noise and limited scalability issues. As a result, most current applications are proof-of-concept or run on quantum simulators rather than true quantum processors [20]. The distance between theoretical quantum computing and practical implementation decreases rapidly as development occurs in quantum error correction and hardware production together with software improvements. Quantum computing and AI can unite to create biological system simulation in real time and exact drug-receptor dynamics modeling and quick screening of big chemical libraries for a modern computational drug discovery revolution (Figure 9.3).

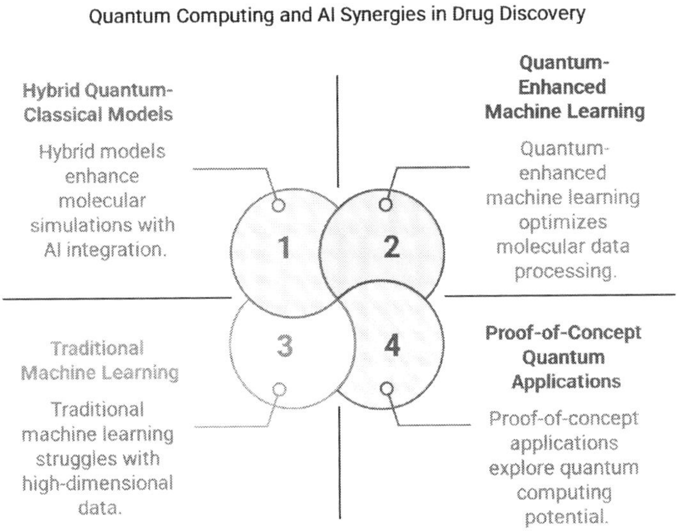

Figure 9.3 Quantum Computing and AI Synergies in Drug Discovery

AI in Personalized and Precision Medicine

AI-Driven Patient Stratification and Polypharmacology Modeling

Precision medicine delivers targeted therapeutic medicine according to individual biological and environmental variations together with lifestyle aspects. AI excels at patient stratification because it examines extensive datasets composed of genomic and proteomic and metabolomic and clinical information to detect particular patient groups who would benefit from specific treatments. ML algorithms can uncover hidden patterns and correlations across complex data, enabling more accurate classification of disease phenotypes and predicting therapeutic efficacy [21]. The capability of AI to model polypharmacology allows researchers to find drugs that address multiple targets especially for diseases, such as cancer and neurodegenerative disorders, that do not respond well to single-drug therapy.

Use of AI in Designing Patient-Specific Therapies

The incorporation of AI technology in drug design enables treatment strategies that deliver highly personalized care to patients on a previously unreachable magnitude. AI tools evaluate individual patient information comprising genetic fault patterns and biological indicator data along with disease markers which guides the identification of new drugs or existing drug modifications. NLP tools can mine scientific literature and EHRs to match patient profiles with potential treatments [22]. With support from AI systems healthcare providers gain the capability to locate blend treatment approaches that maximize individual treatment results alongside minimal adverse response patterns (Table 9.3).

Table 9.3 AI in Personalized and Precision Medicine

Application	*AI Approach*	*Key Benefits*	*Challenges*
Patient Stratification	Machine Learning, NLP	Identification of subgroups of patients with similar treatment responses	Data privacy, the complexity of integrating diverse data types.
Polypharmacology Modeling	Graph Neural Networks (GNNs)	Understanding interactions between multiple drug targets	Addressing drug-drug interactions and polypharmacy.
Patient-Specific Therapies	Deep Learning, Reinforcement Learning	Designing tailored therapies based on individual genetic makeup	Data heterogeneity and small sample sizes.
Digital Twins	AI and Simulation Models	Simulating patient responses to drugs before clinical use	Ensuring model accuracy and reliability.

Digital Twins in Drug Discovery and Response Prediction

Precision medicine saw a fundamental shift with the advent of "digital twins" which represent patients through AI-manipulated real-world healthcare information. Electronic copies of patients can display disease evolution as well as test treatment responses while showing expected intervention results. In drug discovery, digital twins can be used to test thousands of therapeutic strategies in silico before selecting the most promising ones for clinical trials, thereby reducing time and cost. This technology juts in with ongoing health monitoring processes that help healthcare professionals adjust treatment regimens as therapy needs evolve [23]. Digital twins will establish themselves as foundational elements for personalizing therapies and clinical choices in future healthcare practices because of developing data collection capabilities and enhanced predictive models.

AI in Vaccine Development and Infectious Disease Management

Role of AI in Epitope Prediction and Immunogenicity Modeling

Research indicates that AI demonstrates remarkable capability for predicting epitopes which are small pathogenic fragments that generate immune responses when vaccine development requires such prediction. Large immunological datasets undergo ML algorithmic evaluation in order to discover insolvent viral or bacterial sequences which generate robust immune reactions. This process, known as epitope prediction, traditionally required time-consuming laboratory experiments, but AI models can now predict epitopes with high accuracy based on the structure and sequence of pathogens [24]. Immunogenicity modeling functions together with AI technology to model immune system responses against different antigenic elements for designing optimized vaccines which also demonstrate better safety characteristics.

Accelerated Vaccine Design (e.g., mRNA Platform Optimization)

AI stands essential in accelerated vaccine development by focusing on optimization of mRNA vaccine platforms that resulted in fast COVID-19 vaccine production. ML algorithms support the selection of optimal antigen sequences that mRNA strands need. These algorithms can also optimize delivery mechanisms, such as lipid nanoparticles, to ensure stability and efficient uptake by human cells. In the case of mRNA vaccines, AI can model the stability and expression of mRNA in various cell types, predict potential immunogenicity issues, and fine-tune the formulation to maximize efficacy [25]. The AI-powered optimization technology provides enhanced vaccine development speed along with enlarged production capacities for current infectious disease vaccines and future vaccine development.

Pandemic Preparedness with AI Surveillance Systems

The development of trained AI systems now helps nations establish better pandemic reaction capabilities through the implementation of advanced monitoring methods. AI algorithms identify emerging infectious disease outbreaks in real time through their analysis of health records data and social media and travel pattern information as well as environmental sensor data. Such surveillance systems monitor pathogen genetic changes while saving healthcare professionals the ability to project disease spread patterns and detect pandemic risks. In addition, AI can integrate this surveillance data with predictive modeling to forecast the course of an outbreak, optimize containment strategies, and allocate resources efficiently [26]. AI-powered systems help public health authorities take more effective steps against infectious diseases while giving them the essential resources to minimize the duration it takes to create countermeasures starting from pathogen discovery until vaccine or antiviral therapy development.

Federated Learning and Data Privacy in AI Drug Discovery

Challenges of Data Centralization in Pharmaceutical Research

The traditional pharmaceutical research process gathers extensive sensitive patient data along with proprietary datasets at a single centralized location for evaluation purposes. While this approach can foster collaborative research, it introduces significant challenges, particularly regarding data privacy, security, and regulatory compliance. Patient information as well as intellectual property remains at risk of privacy breaches through attacks on centralized datasets. The General Data Protection Regulation (GDPR) implemented by the European Union along with other global regulations control how personal data uses and storage operations must be managed [27]. These challenges create roadblocks for cross-institutional and international collaboration, hindering the progress of AI-driven drug discovery. The centralization process has the potential to create biased datasets since some patient populations and different geographic areas fail to be represented within the system.

Federated and Decentralized AI Frameworks

AI model training becomes possible through federated learning alongside decentralized AI frameworks because these systems eliminate the requirement to move sensitive information to central storage places. In a federated learning setup, multiple institutions or organizations train ML models locally on their own data and share only the model updates (such as gradients) rather than the raw data. The approach enables companies to build potent collaborative AI models which fulfill data privacy standards and privacy regulations. Decentralized AI systems grant researchers opportunities to work together on dispersed datasets spanning multiple institutions as well as regions or international boundaries without compromising privacy or security protocols [28]. These frameworks foster a more inclusive approach to drug discovery by ensuring that diverse and geographically representative datasets are used for model development, while simultaneously safeguarding sensitive health and genetic information.

Secure Multi-Party Computation (SMPC) in Model Training

Secure Multi-Party Computation (SMPC) protects decentralized AI systems together with federated learning through its cryptographic capabilities which stop every participant from accessing others' confidential information. SMPC functions as an AI drug discovery mechanism that enables pharmaceutical companies, hospitals along with research institutions to build AI models jointly while maintaining complete privacy on all proprietary information. Through SMPC, the raw data never leaves the local storage of any participant, and computations are performed on encrypted data. The results are then aggregated and shared in a way that protects the confidentiality of individual datasets. Model training security relies on this approach which meets data privacy laws to become a vital tool for AI pharmaceutical research that handles sensitive health-related information [29]. SMPC technology shows the potential to completely change pharmaceutical company and research organization collaboration regarding drug discovery efforts while upholding data secrecy.

Regulatory and Ethical Considerations

Transparency and Explainability of AI Decisions

For AI systems employed in drug discovery and development laboratories, it is essential to maintain complete transparency of AI decision-making processes particularly when working in clinical or regulatory frameworks. AI models, particularly DL algorithms, often operate as "black boxes," where the decision-making process is not easily interpretable by humans. The absence of explainable decision-making processes creates worries about trust and safety as well as accountability particularly when applied to medically crucial situations. Public and healthcare entities together with regulatory agencies demand full understanding regarding the AI processes that impact patient results as well as community health. The implementation of transparent AI approaches should reveal the information about both data processing methods and predictive mechanisms as well as the reasons guiding particular outcome results [30]. This ensures that AI-based decisions are not only scientifically valid but also ethically sound, enabling stakeholders to verify, challenge, and improve those decisions when necessary.

Regulatory Frameworks and Validation (FDA, EMA Perspectives)

The U.S. Food and Drug Administration (FDA) together with the European Medicines Agency (EMA) have recently established regulatory frameworks to validate AI-based drug discovery tools regarding safety and both efficiency and regulatory compliance standards. The regulatory bodies of the FDA and EMA have developed standards which AI drug development models need to fulfill in order to demonstrate scientific reliability together with valid results. For instance, the FDA's Software as a Medical Device (SaMD) framework outlines the criteria for regulatory approval of AI applications, focusing on the clinical safety and performance of the AI tool in real-world settings [31]. The EMA requires manufacturers to implement strong validation tests with solid clinical performance tests following market release while continuing ongoing system monitoring after deployment. The implementation frameworks operate as vital components to guarantee both safety and performance of AI tools that serve drug discovery and personalized medicine functions. However, the evolving nature of AI technology presents challenges for regulatory bodies to stay ahead of rapid advancements while ensuring patient protection.

Addressing Bias, Reproducibility, and Accountability

The main drawback of AI drug discovery stems from data sources that introduce unintentional biases into algorithm training. AI models developed from non-diverse and biased training sets create faulty predictions that lead to faulty results which affect specific patient groups in an unjust manner. Dealing with bias needs training datasets to contain broad diversity which includes all populations worldwide and employs detection and mitigation systems during model construction. Reproducibility is another critical issue research findings must be replicable, especially in the context of AI-driven discoveries, where different research teams should be able to obtain similar results using the same AI models. Complete model transparency enables clear algorithm documentation and independent data-code verification necessitates sharing both datasets and programming source codes [32]. The most important aspect in this situation is making sure responsible parties remain accountable especially when AI systems determine critical healthcare decisions. Clear guidelines must be established for who is responsible if an AI-driven decision leads to harm or failure, whether it be the developers, the pharmaceutical companies, or healthcare providers. AI drug discovery will develop thanks to regulatory and ethical standards which ensure its ethical and fair use in upcoming years.

Future Outlook and Emerging Paradigms

AI in Automated Closed-Loop Drug Discovery Labs

Drug discovery approaches face a major transformation because automated closed-loop systems are entering the market to integrate AI throughout drug development processes. A system will unite high-throughput screening components with real-time data analytic procedures and autonomous decision engines to create a closed-loop drug discovery platform which runs continuously through the product evaluation cycle [33]. AI will be able to automate the design of molecules, predict their properties, and simulate biological interactions in silico, thereby reducing the time and cost associated with traditional drug discovery methods. The automated systems help drug discovery through faster development alongside enhanced precision by automatically refining hypotheses and adapt models with experimental data to autonomously create new drug candidates. The integration of robotics, AI, and ML will transform drug discovery from a manual, labor-intensive process into a highly efficient and intelligent operation, dramatically accelerating the timeline for developing new therapeutics [34].

Human-AI Collaboration and Cognitive Augmentation

AI in drug discovery is expected to partner with humans to produce enhanced collaborative capabilities rather than seeking to substitute expert pharmaceutical knowledge. AI operates as an essential breakthrough technology that enables researchers to handle extensive data volumes and detect subtle patterns along with generating research directions. In this context, AI will act as a cognitive augmentation system, enhancing the abilities of researchers by providing them with insights and hypotheses that can drive experimentation. Researchers collaborating with AI will tap into AI computational strength and data management capabilities as they use their domain experience along with imaginative thinking to understand the outcomes produced by the system. This collaboration will enable scientists to focus on higher-level decision-making and innovative strategies, while AI tackles repetitive tasks, such as data analysis, pattern recognition, and predictive modeling [35]. Drug design innovation will arise from human-AI synergies to enable researchers to investigate previously unknown concepts in molecular medicine.

Potential for AGI (Artificial General Intelligence) in Molecular Medicine

Artificial General Intelligence (AGI) in molecular medicine has outstanding potential to successfully revolutionize drug discovery practices and healthcare delivery through advanced developments in the future. The capabilities of machines capable of executing intellectual tasks human beings can do (known as AGI) within drug discovery will achieve completely new drug discovery heights. An AGI system would not be limited to narrow tasks, such as predicting molecular properties or analyzing data but would be capable of synthesizing vast amounts of medical, biological, and chemical knowledge to propose innovative therapies and even create new classes of drugs autonomously [36]. With simulations of complex biological systems that existing AI lacks the ability to perform AGI can effectively predict drug interactions in addition to side effects and prolonged outcomes using precise calculations. The future of molecular medicine depends on AGI's capability to duplicate human intellectual skills for connecting information between scientific fields which leads to innovative treatments for diseases without pharmaceutical remedies. However, while AGI offers immense promise, its development comes with significant challenges, including ensuring safety, ethical considerations, and control over decision-making processes. Advancements in AGI for molecular medicine would transform drug development capabilities by creating more effective methods to discover and tailor medication solutions, thus establishing novel standards for healthcare progress [37].

Conclusion

Summary of Current Advancements and Visionary Trends

AI transformations in drug discovery have evolved from basic analysis instruments into powerful predictive models which find applications in molecular behavior forecasting and drug optimization along with new treatment discovery. Modern advances in AI drug discovery have enhanced the entire pharmaceutical pipeline starting from the discovery of targets through lead development into clinical studies using DL and generative algorithms and RL methods. Cutting-edge tools like AlphaFold for protein structure prediction, deep generative models for drug design, and AI-powered platforms for personalized medicine are transforming the way we approach drug discovery, with potential applications ranging from infectious diseases to cancer therapies [38]. The upcoming future of molecular medicine can be predicted through advancements like integrated AI discovery systems utilizing closed-loop functionality and quantum model advancements and the possibility of AGI. The improved drug development speed and efficiency brought by recent advancements enables the development of solutions for complex precision medicine challenges and the improvement of global health services and individualized treatments.

Key Takeaways for Academia, Industry, and Policymakers

Academic institutions gain new possibilities for advancing their study of ML together with bioinformatics and computational biology as part of AI drug discovery integration. Drug discovery success through AI depends on frequent teamwork between pharmacologists, biologists and computational scientists so academic institutions must establish interdisciplinary training for future researchers. Industry players, particularly pharmaceutical companies, should embrace AI technologies to streamline drug discovery and reduce the associated costs and time [39]. The drug industry must keep prioritizing AI model transparency to implement these systems properly within drug development processes. Policymakers must recognize the transformative potential of AI and establish frameworks that encourage innovation while addressing ethical concerns, data privacy, and regulatory hurdles. Global collaboration must establish standards which guarantee safe ethical usage of AI healthcare systems since AI systems are becoming increasingly autonomous when making decisions.

Strategic Roadmap for Sustainable AI Integration

Drug discovery needs strategic planning to achieve sustainable AI implementation. Academic institutions alongside industrial organizations must dedicate financial support toward AI scholarly activities to develop competent professionals. Implementing training programs that unite experts from different fields will create connections between algorithm-based techniques and typical drug development approaches. AI platforms need to include design features which ensure they are flexible and able to process variable amounts of data as research demands evolve. It is also crucial to address the challenges of data privacy, especially with patient-specific data, and to develop decentralized frameworks, such as federated learning, that allow for secure, privacy-preserving AI applications [40]. A changing regulatory infrastructure needs to track technological growth in order to guarantee medical validation for AI models that healthcare staff and research scholars trust. Above all else, ethical standards must lead AI implementation efforts to maintain transparent systems which are bias-free while being accountable especially for highly sensitive applications in personalized medicine and drug price determination. We will construct a worldwide platform where AI-driven drug discovery gets speed-ups while ensuring fair access to lifesaving therapeutics through strong partnerships along with funded AI systems and established compliance frameworks focused on safety and fairness in use.

References

1. Service, R. F. (2024). AI tools set off an explosion of designer proteins. *Science*, *386*, 260–261.
2. Callaway, E. (2024). Chemistry Nobel goes to developers of AlphaFold AI that predicts protein structures. *Nature*, *634*, 525–526.
3. Fu, L., Shi, S., & Yi, J., et al. (2024). ADMETlab 3.0: An updated comprehensive online ADMET prediction platform enhanced with broader coverage, improved performance, API functionality and decision support. *Nucleic Acids Research*, *52*(W1), W422–W431.
4. Aminabee, S. K., Prabhakar, M. C., Prasad, R. G. S. V., & Lakshmana Rao, A. (2011). Screening the pharmacological activity of cerium oxide nanoparticles in-vitro. *Biomedical and Pharmacology Journal*, *4*(2), 287–289.
5. Chakravarty, K., Antontsev, V., & Bundey, Y., et al. (2021). Driving success in personalized medicine through AI-enabled computational modeling. *Drug Discovery Today*, *26*, 1459–1465.
6. Lourenço, M. P., Hostaš, J., & Bellinger, C., et al. (2024). Reinforcement learning for *in silico* determination of adsorbate-substrate structures. *Journal of Computational Chemistry*, *45*, 1289–1302.

7. Zhavoronkov, A., Ivanenkov, Y. A., & Aliper, A., et al. (2019). Deep learning enables rapid identification of potent DDR1 kinase inhibitors. *Nature Biotechnology*, *37*, 1038–1040.
8. Guerrero, M., Urbano, M., & Kim, E. K., et al. (2019). Design and synthesis of a novel and selective kappa opioid receptor (KOR) antagonist (BTRX-335140). *Journal of Medicinal Chemistry*, *62*(4), 1761–1780.
9. Aminabee, S. K., Lakshmana Rao, A., Sowmya, K., Nymisha, D., Kusuma Naga Lakshmi, K., Manikanta, K. V. N. S., & Praveen Kumar, P. (2019). Evaluation of analgesic activity of *Ficus palmata*. *Iranian Journal of Pharmaceutical Sciences*, *15*(3), 47–60.
10. Plas, S., Pircher, A., & Heidegger, I. (2023). Pembrolizumab in mCRPC-combination therapies as breakthrough to success? *Current Opinion in Urology*, *33*(5), 458–471.
11. Jones, J. D., Rajachandran, L., & Yocca, F., et al. (2023). Sublingual dexmedetomidine (BXCL501) reduces opioid withdrawal symptoms: Findings from a multi-site, phase 1b/2, randomized, double-blind, placebo-controlled trial. *American Journal of Drug and Alcohol Abuse*, *49*(1), 109–122.
12. Aminabee, S. K., Lakshmana Rao, A., & Chinna Eswaraiah, M. (2020). In-vivo antioxidant activity of different fractions of *Indigofera barberi* against paracetamol-induced toxicity in rats. *Turkish Journal of Pharmaceutical Sciences*, *17*(2), 136–140.
13. Lacouture, M. E., Dion, H., & Ravipaty, S., et al. (2021). A phase I safety study of topical calcitriol (BPM31543) for the prevention of chemotherapy-induced alopecia. *Breast Cancer Research and Treatment*, *186*(1), 107–114.
14. Varkaris, A., Pazolli, E., & Gunaydin, H., et al. (2024). Discovery and clinical proof-of-concept of RLY-2608, a first-in-class mutant-selective allosteric PI3Kα inhibitor. *Cancer Discovery*, *14*(2), 240–257.
15. Kyriakidis, F., Kogias, D., & Venou, T. M., et al. (2023). Updated perspectives on the diagnosis and management of familial adenomatous polyposis. *Applied Clinical Genetics*, *16*, 139–153.
16. Prasanth, D. S. N. B. K., Aminabee, S. K., Lakshmana Rao, A., Teja, N., Bhargavi, K., Monika, C., Pujitha, B., Sandhya, T., Lalitha, A., & Siva Prasad, P. (2020). Anthelmintic activity of *Mansoa alliacea* against *Pheretima posthuma*: In-vitro and in-silico approach. *Thai Journal of Pharmaceutical Sciences*, *4*(3), 186–196.
17. Giammarile, F., Paez, D., & Zimmermann, R., et al. (2024). Production and regulatory issues for theranostics. *The Lancet Oncology*, *25*(6), e260–e269.
18. Jumper, J., Evans, R., & Pritzel, A., et al. (2021). Applying and improving AlphaFold at CASP14. *Proteins: Structure, Function, and Bioinformatics*, *89*(12), 1711–1721.
19. Prasanth, D. S. N. B. K., Aminabee, S. K., Lakshmana Rao, A., Guntupalli, C., Reddy, A. R., Kulandaivelu, U., Rao, S. N. K., & Rajeshwari, P. (2021). Inhibitory effects of *Mansoa alliacea* in Freund's adjuvant arthritis on inflammatory markers and its confirmation by in-silico strategy. *Thai Journal of Pharmaceutical Sciences*, *45*(6), 532–544.
20. Li, S., Peng, L., & Chen, L., et al. (2024). Discovery of highly bioactive peptides through hierarchical structural information and molecular dynamics simulations. *Journal of Chemical Information and Modeling*, *64*(4), 8164–8175.
21. Segler, M. H. S., Preuss, M., & Waller, M. P. (2018). Planning chemical syntheses with deep neural networks and symbolic AI. *Nature*, *555*, 604–610.
22. Aminabee, S. K., Santhi Krupa, D., Hanumanth Rao, K., Sirisha, V., Anitha Kumari, V., Nagasen, D., Sujiya, B., & Leelavati, T. S. (2023). Pharmacoeconomic analysis of biologic vs. biosimilar therapies in rheumatoid arthritis. *International Journal of Chemical and Biochemical Sciences*, *24*(4), 395–400.
23. Schoenmaker, L., Béquignon, O. J. M., & Jespers, W., et al. (2023). UnCorrupt SMILES: A novel approach to de novo design. *Journal of Cheminformatics*, *15*, 22.
24. Ucak, U. V., Ashyrmamatov, I., & Lee, J. (2023). Reconstruction of lossless molecular representations from fingerprints. *Journal of Cheminformatics*, *15*, 26.

25. Kutsal, M., Ucar, F., & Kati, N. (2024). Computational drug discovery on human immunodeficiency virus with a customized long short-term memory variational autoencoder deep-learning architecture. *CPT: Pharmacometrics & Systems Pharmacology*, *13*, 308–316.
26. Leelavati, T. S., Madhavi, S., Kamal, G., Raju, P. V. M., Susmitha, K., Vinod, M., & Aminabee, S. K. (2023). Revolutionizing healthcare delivery: Telemedicine's influence on access and patient satisfaction. *International Journal of Chemical and Biochemical Sciences*, *24*(5), 106–115.
27. Nehal, M., Khatoon, J., & Akhtar, S., et al. (2024). Computational insights into inhibiting EphA2: Integrating structure-based virtual screening, docking, and molecular dynamics simulations for small molecule discovery. *Cellular and Molecular Biology*, *70*, 16–31.
28. Shen, C., Hu, X., & Gao, J., et al. (2021). The impact of cross-docked poses on performance of machine learning classifier for protein-ligand binding pose prediction. *Journal of Cheminformatics*, *13*, 81.
29. Aminabee, S. K., Devi Mallika, K., & Lakshmana Rao, A. (2023). Natural resources in management and treatment of diseases: A review. *Pharma Times*, *55*(11), 7–10.
30. Zhang, Y., Wang, M., & Zhang, E., et al. (2024). Artificial intelligence in the screening, diagnosis, and management of aortic stenosis. *Reviews in Cardiovascular Medicine*, *25*, 31.
31. Zhang, X., Shen, C., & Zhang, H., et al. (2024). Advancing ligand docking through deep learning: Challenges and prospects in virtual screening. *Accounts of Chemical Research*, *57*, 1500–1509.
32. Aminabee, S. K., & Lakshmana Rao, A. (2024). Computational identification of selected bioactive compounds from *Cedrus deodara* as inhibitors against SARS-CoV-2 main protease: A pharmacoinformatics study. *Indian Drugs*, *61*(2), 78–91.
33. Gantenbein, L., Cerminara, S. E., & Maul, J. T., et al. (2024). Artificial intelligence-driven skin aging simulation as a novel skin cancer prevention. *Dermatology*, *241*(1), 1–13.
34. Clarke, B., Holtkamp, E., & Öztürk, H., et al. (2024). Integration of variant annotations using deep set networks boosts rare variant association testing. *Nature Genetics*, *56*, 2271–2280.
35. Pogodin, P. V., Salina, E. G., & Semenov, V. V. et al. (2024). Ligand-based virtual screening and biological evaluation of inhibitors of *Mycobacterium tuberculosis* H37Rv. *SAR and QSAR in Environmental Research*, *35*, 53–69.
36. Ravi Shankar, K., Aminabee, S. K., Ramana, G., Chenchu Lakshmi, K. N. V., & Indusree, G. (2024). Formulation and evaluation of propranolol hydrochloride floating tablets by 32 factorial design. *International Journal of Drug Delivery Technology*, *14*(4), 2060–2067.
37. Kumar, V., Jangid, K., & Kumar, N., et al. (2024). 3D-QSAR-based pharmacophore modelling of quinazoline derivatives for the identification of acetylcholinesterase inhibitors through virtual screening, molecular docking, molecular dynamics and DFT studies. *Journal of Biomolecular Structure and Dynamics*, *43*, 1–15.
38. Krishnan, K. A., Valavi, S. G., & Joy, A. (2024). Identification of novel EGFR inhibitors for the targeted therapy of colorectal cancer using pharmacophore modelling, docking, molecular dynamic simulation and biological activity prediction. *Anti-Cancer Agents in Medicinal Chemistry*, *24*, 263–279.
39. Ghasemi, F., Fassihi, A., & Pérez-Sánchez, H., et al. (2017). The role of different sampling methods in improving biological activity prediction using deep belief network. *Journal of Computational Chemistry*, *38*, 195–203.
40. Minnich, A. J., McLoughlin, K., & Tse, M., et al. (2020). AMPL: A data-driven modeling pipeline for drug discovery. *Journal of Chemical Information and Modeling*, *60*(4), 1955–1968.

10 Practical Applications and Strategies for Implementation

Introduction

AI's Transformative Role in Medication Research

The adoption of Artificial Intelligence (AI) throughout pharmaceutical and biomedical research produces significant changes to the modern medication discovery and testing processes along with market release stages. AI enables researchers to access automated tools which allow them to analyze data effectively and create biological system models and make precise clinical outcome predictions. Techniques, such as machine learning, deep learning, and natural language processing, are now capable of screening vast chemical libraries, identifying promising drug candidates, and even repurposing existing drugs for new therapeutic uses. The reduction of drug discovery timelines together with optimized resource allocation and personalized medicine representation makes AI an indispensable asset for modern pipelines in drug development [1].

Need for Practical Frameworks and Actionable Strategies

The successful application of AI in drug research requires dealing with actual obstacles that stand in its way of achieving significant progress. Cortical organizations encounter multiple obstacles during workflow transition from theoretical models because they must solve data differences and staffing issues and unclear rules and experimental-computational segregation. Furthermore, the pharmaceutical domain has traditionally been slow to adopt disruptive technologies due to concerns over validation, interpretability, and safety. Organizations require pressing frameworks which cover both operational execution together with strategic development and ethical rules in addition to collaborative models. These framework systems protect the scalability alongside reliability of AI technologies and maintain consistency with scientific requirements and regulatory standards [2].

DOI: 10.4324/9781003616177-10

Objectives of the Chapter

This chapter serves as a guide to bridge the divide between AI theory and its successful, responsible application in the field of medication research. It sets out to achieve the following objectives [3]:

- An analysis of current AI technology applications in pharmaceutical research is provided through examination of new discoveries and experimental studies.
- To outline practical methods and tools that facilitate the integration of AI into drug discovery and development workflows, including strategies for model validation, data preprocessing, and interpretation of outputs.
- Standard operating procedures (SOPs) and best practices based approaches will enable consistent and reproducible and compliant operation of AI-driven research.
- To explore collaborative frameworks that enable effective synergy between AI experts, biologists, chemists, clinicians, and regulatory professionals.
- The assessment includes risk identification together with data security improvements and bias correction in algorithms and AI prediction limitation strategies (Figure 10.1).

Framework for AI Integration in Medication Research

Mapping AI across Drug Discovery and Development Stages

The integration of AI at strategic positions along the drug development lifecycle helps to boost efficiency rates as well as lower errors and enhance decision-making capabilities. Modern pharmaceutical development processes across every stage receive fundamental advantages through the data-based perceptions of AI systems [4].

Target Identification and Validation

AI algorithms, particularly machine learning (ML) and deep learning models, have revolutionized the process of identifying and validating drug targets. AI uses three data types, including genomics, transcriptomics, proteomics, to discover disease-specific molecular pathways. Natural language processing techniques help scientists extract new target discoveries by examining scientific literature through computers and clinical databases with automated methods. This accelerates the identification process while improving the likelihood of target relevance and druggability.

Compound Screening and Optimization

Traditional high-throughput screening (HTS) is time-consuming and resource-intensive. Virtual screening enhanced through AI makes it possible to predict the

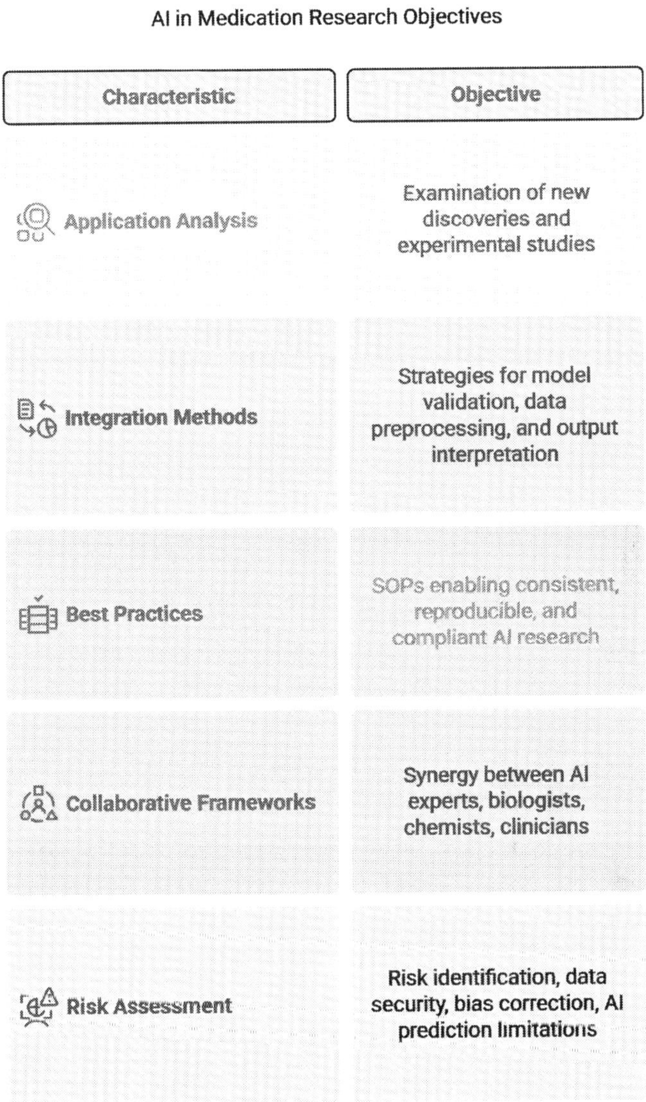

Figure 10.1 AI in Medication Research Objectives

biological properties of numerous compounds before physical experimentation. The combination of reinforcement learning algorithms and generative modeling approaches, including GANs or variational autoencoders (VAEs) produces enhanced molecules through an optimization process to attain optimal potency along with selectivity and pharmacokinetic characteristics [5]. AI tools also facilitate Structure-Activity Relationship (SAR) modeling, enabling iterative optimization cycles based on predictive analytics.

Preclinical and Clinical Trial Design

AI supports rational design of both preclinical studies and clinical trials. The application of AI technology in animal experiments predicts the toxicity levels and bioavailability and off-target effects through minimal experimental data collection. AI enables medical research by dividing patient populations, recruiting participants and tracking them through analysis of electronic health records (EHRs), genomics, wearable sensors, and other health databases. Predictive models can anticipate trial outcomes or identify biomarkers correlated with therapeutic efficacy, thereby reducing attrition rates [6].

Pharmacovigilance and Post-Marketing Surveillance

The detection of both uncommon side effects and extended-term adverse drug reactions becomes essential after drugs obtain market approval. The analysis of large quantities of real-world data using AI produces safety signal detection that happens earlier than traditional methods do. Algorithmic programs collect relevant information from non-structured document texts through NLP tools and anomaly detection methods detect patterns requiring examination. This strengthens regulatory compliance and enhances patient safety (Table 10.1).

Utilizing Implementation Science for AI Adoption

The combination of AI theoretical potential for drug development work has been acknowledged but successful daily implementation demands proper adoption strategies. The interdisciplinary field of implementation science provides tools and methodologies to make necessary improvements in the use of innovations through routine practice [7].

By applying implementation frameworks, such as the Consolidated Framework for Implementation Research (CFIR) or Reach, Effectiveness, Adoption, Implementation, and Maintenance (RE-AIM), pharmaceutical organizations can:

- Workers need to evaluate all relevant organizational aspects for readiness like staff knowledge levels and infrastructure and work environment cultural elements.

Table 10.1 Stages of Drug Discovery and AI Integration Points

Stage of Drug Development	*AI Application*	*Tools/Techniques Used*
Target Identification and Validation	Gene-disease association, pathway mapping	ML, NLP, BioBERT
Compound Screening and Optimization	Predicting bioactivity, ADMET properties	DeepChem, generative models
Preclinical and Clinical Trial Design	Patient stratification, outcome prediction	Predictive analytics, simulation tools
Pharmacovigilance	Detecting adverse events, risk signal detection	NLP on EHRs and social media, ML algorithms
Post-Marketing Surveillance	Real-world evidence analysis, continuous safety monitoring	AI dashboards, anomaly detection systems

- Engineers should implement AI solutions according to individual workflows to achieve user-friendly interfaces that scientists and clinical staff will adopt.
- Address barriers, such as data privacy concerns, algorithm transparency, and regulatory uncertainty [8].
- Performance evaluation should be based on specific metrics that measure clinical achievements and end-user satisfaction together with cost-effectiveness.

Technological Infrastructure and Tools

The successful deployment of AI for medication research depends completely upon establishing strong technological infrastructure. System success demands advanced AI model technology and optimized platforms and computing systems which effectively process large biomedical datasets. In this section, we explore the AI technologies actively used in drug discovery and development, the software tools that enable their deployment, and the computational requirements necessary for their successful execution [9].

AI Models in Practice

Machine Learning (ML) and Deep Learning (DL)

The pharmacokinetic process uses support vector machines together with random forests and gradient boosting algorithms from Machine Learning to predict toxicity levels and compound effectiveness. The AI subdomain called Deep Learning delivers exceptional capabilities for analyzing complex patterns between numerous components which appear within biomedical datasets, including sequence data and imaging and biochemical structures [10]. DL architectures like convolutional neural networks (CNNs) and recurrent neural networks (RNNs) have shown great promise in predicting molecular behavior and classifying medical data.

Natural Language Processing (NLP) for Electronic Health Records (EHRs)

NLP techniques automatically extract and interpret unstructured medical content found in clinical notes as well as medical literature along with EHRs. Research scientists can gain meaningful findings from large biomedical document sets through BioBERT (Bidirectional Encoder Representations from Transformers for Biomedical Text Mining) which enables clinical hypothesis discovery and trial improvement [11].

Generative AI for Molecular Design

The molecular discovery process gets a revolutionary transformation from two AI models classified under generative AI: VAEs and Generative Adversarial Networks (GANs). The system develops new chemical structures through automatic learning from present compound data collections which possess preferred pharmaceutical properties. This accelerates the identification of lead molecules with enhanced specificity, solubility, and stability profiles [12].

Platforms and Software

AlphaFold

DeepMind produced AlphaFold as the technology that changed the way AI predicts protein structures. AlphaFold achieves precise mappings of amino acid sequence folds, which leads scientists to understand protein interactions and functions as a requirement for structure-based drug development.

IBM Watson for Drug Discovery

IBM Watson powered by AI and cognitive computing supplies researchers with help to discover drug targets as well as biomarkers and therapeutic strategies. The system performs two types of data analysis by evaluating structured clinical databases while also processing unstructured scientific text to generate expert recommendations [13].

DeepChem

DeepChem is an open-source Python library that bridges cheminformatics and machine learning. The software offers capabilities for developing neural network systems which focus on quantum chemistry work as well as molecular property estimations and virtual screening tasks, thus enabling users to create efficient prototype models swiftly.

BioBERT

BioBERT exists as a biomedical text-focused domain-specific language model that received training on big biomedical text databases [1]. BioBERT exhibits its most beneficial properties for three essential biomedical operations which are text classification and both named entity recognition (NER) and relation extraction functions, thus serving outstandingly well in drug repurposing research and literature mining activities (Figure 10.2).

AI Platforms and Software Comparison

Characteristic	AlphaFold	IBM Watson	DeepChem	BioBERT
Primary Function	Protein structure prediction	Drug discovery assistance	Cheminformatics and ML	Biomedical text analysis
Technology	Deep learning AI	AI and cognitive computing	Open-source Python library	Domain-specific language model
Application	Structure-based drug development	Drug target and biomarker discovery	Quantum chemistry and virtual screening	Drug repurposing and literature mining

Figure 10.2 AI Platforms and Software Comparison

Cloud Computing and High-Performance Computing Requirements

The extensive data availability together with complicated AI model requirements surpass the capabilities of traditional computing systems used for drug research through AI. Organizations can access scalable on-demand computing services through high-performance computing (HPC) together with cloud solutions operating from Amazon Web Services (AWS), Google Cloud, and Microsoft Azure platform [14]. These platforms allow:

- Parallel processing of datasets for faster training of AI models.
- Secure storage and sharing of sensitive biomedical and clinical data.
- The system supports AI/ML frameworks TensorFlow, PyTorch, and Scikit-learn to perform model development then deployment.

Best Practices for Implementation

Organizations seeking successful implementation of AI as a pharmaceutical research and development tool must follow established strategic best practices. Such best practices enable AI tools to work reliably with valid outcomes while fulfilling all regulatory requirements. Key focus areas include the integrity of data, transparency of algorithms, rigorous model validation, and the use of agile methodologies to streamline deployment.

Data Curation and Quality Control

Medication research generally depends on data which is of premier quality and thoroughly annotated. Data imperfections, such as inconsistencies or incompleteness or noisiness, cause results to become either erroneous or invalid. The process of data curation includes thorough systematic methods for cleaning biomedical datasets along with labeling and format modification and validation of chemical libraries and clinical trial records and EHR datasets [2].

Best practices include:

- Establishing standardized data ontologies and formats (e.g., CDISC and HL7).
- Removing duplicate or irrelevant records.
- Ensuring balanced datasets to avoid algorithmic bias.
- Regular auditing and updating of datasets to reflect current medical knowledge.

Explainable AI (XAI) for Regulatory Compliance

Complex drug development with AI needs to pass rigorous government standards for ensuring product safety as well as regulatory compliance. AI systems with explainable decision-making capability referred to as XAI deliver transparent and interpretable insights about their processes [3].

In medication research:

- XAI helps justify model predictions in clinical contexts (e.g., adverse effect prediction or compound prioritization).
- The Shapley Additive Explanations (SHAP) and Local Interpretable Model-Agnostic Explanations (LIME) methods enable tracking of input variables that affect AI predictive outcomes.
- Transparency builds trust among stakeholders and is often a prerequisite for regulatory approval by agencies like the FDA or EMA.

Model Validation and Reproducibility in Drug Discovery Pipelines

Rigorous validation is essential for AI models to gain credibility and usability in real-world drug discovery [15]. This involves:

- Splitting data into training, validation, and test sets.
- The evaluation of generalizability requires both cross-validation and external validation cohorts.
- Benchmarking models against traditional statistical methods and existing drug discovery tools.
- The system requires complete documentation of AI scripts along with evidence tracking for data origin and analytical results recording for reproducible results.

The rise of AI in clinical settings requires independent verification of its results for critical study and medication development applications according to regulatory standards.

Agile Methodologies in AI Tool Deployment

AI technology advancement speed requires organizations to use versatile methods for deploying their systems. Agile methodologies have spread across software development teams bringing new methods to AI deployment in pharmaceutical environments [16].

Key agile practices include:

- Incremental development: Breaking down large AI projects into smaller, manageable tasks with rapid iteration cycles.
- Cross-functional teams: Involving data scientists, pharmacologists, clinicians, and regulatory experts from the start.
- Continuous integration and deployment (CI/CD): Automating updates and testing of AI tools in development pipelines.
- Feedback loops: Using stakeholder and end-user input to refine AI models and interfaces regularly (Table 10.2).

Table 10.2 Best Practices for AI Implementation in Drug Discovery

Best Practice	*Purpose*	*Implementation Tip*
Data curation and quality control	Ensure accurate, clean inputs for model training	Use automated data cleaning pipelines
Explainable AI (XAI)	Regulatory transparency and clinical trust	Adopt SHAP, LIME for feature interpretability
Model validation and reproducibility	Scientific robustness	Use standardized benchmarking datasets
Agile methodologies	Fast, iterative deployment of AI models	Employ sprint cycles and user feedback loops

Collaborative Strategies between IT and Pharma Sectors

Building Interdisciplinary Teams

Research integration of AI demands teams consisting of members from multiple scientific fields to bridge different domains of knowledge. Data scientists collaborate with bioinformaticians and pharmacologists and clinicians to form these teams. Data analysis through bioinformatics offers scientists the ability to discover vital relationships between medicines and illnesses. Data scientists and AI engineers design, train, and refine predictive models, while pharmacologists ensure that the data inputs and outputs are grounded in real-world drug behavior. Healthcare professionals offer clinical expertise to help optimize AI systems creating technology solutions that fulfill medical needs [6]. Multiple professionals working together can optimize the deployment of AI technology to enhance drug discovery and development.

Communication and Workflow Alignment

A successful integration of AI through pharmaceutical research areas and clinical settings demands that IT professionals maintain clear communication with pharmacists. The main barrier stems from the need to transform intricate biological issues into computational expressions. For example, identifying drug targets or predicting adverse effects must be reformulated into tasks like classification, regression, or pattern recognition. Shared digital platforms and knowledge bases, such as cloud-based repositories and collaborative workspaces, help facilitate data exchange and joint analysis. Standard vocabularies alongside unified data formats enable field team members to exchange information effectively [17]. Pharmaceutical organizations work with technology organizations spanning from startup companies to global tech giants to trade AI models with data processing abilities along with research materials.

Joint Ventures and Public-Private Partnerships (PPPs)

The rapid spread of AI in pharma production increasingly depends on the formation of public-private partnerships along with joint ventures. AI models and computational resources alongside large-scale datasets undergo partnership-sharing through pharmaceutical technology firm clusters from tech startups to massive global tech companies IMI operates throughout Europe using models like U.S. AMP while establishing partnerships between academic institutions and industries with government regulatory bodies for new scientific research. These partnerships provide access to shared infrastructure, foster transparency in model validation, and facilitate ethical considerations around AI use in healthcare [18]. Moreover, such collaborations often lead to co-development of novel AI platforms and tools tailored specifically for pharmaceutical applications.

Ethical, Legal, and Regulatory Considerations

Handling Patient Data: GDPR, HIPAA, and AI Act Compliance

AI-based medication research relies heavily on accessing big datasets that contain EHRs and genomic information and patient registries. Medical records require both strong data security alongside privacy protection for immediate solution. Every business needs to demonstrate full compliance with European GDPR and United States HIPAA data security protocols in order to use them globally. These laws dictate how data can be collected, stored, shared, and analyzed, emphasizing informed consent, anonymization, and the right to data access and deletion [9]. All healthcare facilities must adhere to European AI Act standards because it requires transparency and establishes risk assessment requirements while requiring accountability for protected data domains.

Bias and Fairness in AI Model Training

The main ethical issue emerges from requiring unbiased training data to develop fair outcome results in AI systems. Any bias found in training datasets used to build AI systems can strengthen or extend current inequalities in healthcare distribution. An AI tool trained using mainly data from a single population subgroup will deliver inferior predictions to other groups so healthcare results become uneven. To mitigate this, data diversity and balance should be prioritized, and fairness metrics must be systematically applied during model development [10]. XAI together with continuous audits allows systems to detect hidden biases, which then enables fairer decision-making throughout drug development and therapy optimization processes.

Regulatory Landscape for AI-Driven Research (FDA, EMA, CDSCO)

The regulatory process which governs AI-assisted drug discovery tools shows active development in present times. Three pharmaceutical regulatory bodies, including FDA, EMA, and CDSCO, are developing guidelines to govern AI applications in healthcare and pharmaceutical sectors. These agencies emphasize the need for transparency, reproducibility, and rigorous validation of AI models used in preclinical and clinical settings. Current regulatory standards recognize AI tools as software-as-a-medical-device (SaMD) requiring three elements – lifecycle management,

Table 10.3 Ethical and Regulatory Guidelines for AI in Pharma

Regulation	*Jurisdiction*	*Purpose*
GDPR	EU	Protects patient data and privacy
HIPAA	USA	Secures health-related personal data
AI Act (proposed)	EU	Classifies AI systems based on risk
FDA/EMA/CDSCO Guidance	Global	Regulates AI/ML tools used in drug development

performance monitoring, and post-market surveillance [19]. Standards-based regulatory frameworks form the entire foundation of worldwide safe innovation development (Table 10.3).

Risk Assessment and Mitigation

Technical Risks: Model Drift, Overfitting, and Generalizability

The reliability and performance of medication research models based on AI systems face numerous technical risks. Model accuracy decreases through model drift which happens when the data distribution modifies over time. Overfitting is another common issue, where a model performs exceptionally well on training data but fails to generalize to new, unseen data. An AI system becomes ineffective when it operates outside its designated range of applicability across therapy areas and between patient groups and research settings [11]. Organizations need to establish model training monitoring and technical vulnerability assessments as essential operational workflows to secure model reliability.

Operational Risks: Resistance, Training, and Integration Challenges

Pharmaceutical workflows face resistance against AI tool adoption due to personnel who do not understand this technology. Staff members doubt the effectiveness of AI technology while worrying about job automation but show minimal willingness to actually implement these systems. Training gaps also hinder smooth implementation, as pharmacologists and clinicians may lack the computational literacy needed to effectively interact with AI systems. The combination of incompatible data formats alongside limited interoperability and obsolete IT systems generates delays and interruptive implementation disruptions [20]. AI implementation succeeds when organizations address these issues through established change management structures alongside open communication pathways.

Risk Mitigation Strategies: Pilot Projects and Phased Rollouts

Organizations should establish pilot programs to evaluate AI tools through real-world testing while managing operational and technical risks. Testing AI models becomes possible in sandbox environments since they recreate operational settings

Table 10.4 Risk Types and Mitigation Strategies

Risk Type	*Example*	*Mitigation Strategy*
Technical	Model drift, overfitting	Continuous model monitoring and re-training
Operational	Resistance to AI adoption, training gaps	Conduct workshops, implement change management
Strategic	Mismatch between tech and clinical goals	Co-develop solutions with domain experts

while keeping actual processes unaffected. Additionally, phased rollouts help to gradually integrate AI tools across departments, ensuring that feedback can be incorporated iteratively [21]. Pharmaceutical organizations can use these methods to decrease operational disruptions and create system reliability while maintaining smooth development of AI-assisted research pipelines (Table 10.4).

Case Studies and Real-World Applications

AI-Driven Drug Repurposing: Lessons from COVID-19

The COVID-19 pandemic created a distinct laboratory for AI implementations to hasten the process of drug reclassification. The entire process employed machine learning algorithms that processed existing drugs alongside clinical trial results and viral proteins to discover promising antiviral candidates. AI platforms, such as BenevolentAI, played a crucial role in identifying baricitinib, a rheumatoid arthritis drug, as a viable treatment for COVID-19, which later gained emergency use authorization [22]. Essential therapy decisions across the world during the pandemic were made possible by fast-paced AI technology development of hypotheses.

Advancing Drug Discovery in Rare Diseases

AI has started entering drug development for rare diseases because both funding and data collection remain sparse for these diseases. AI algorithms use brief datasets containing genetic information to assist teams developing orphan drug targets. For example, AI-driven biomarker identification has improved diagnostic accuracy and facilitated early intervention strategies in conditions like spinal muscular atrophy and Duchenne muscular dystrophy.

Collaborative Success Stories: Pfizer, Novartis, and BenevolentAI

Large pharmaceutical organizations build their AI capabilities through strategic collaboration with other companies. Pfizer established a partnership with IBM Watson to use AI technology for immuno-oncology research that aids in identifying patient outcomes and testing trial approaches. Novartis joined forces with Microsoft to launch an AI innovation lab which works on early stage drug development through deep learning and cloud computing methods [23]. Similarly, BenevolentAI collaborates with various pharma firms, offering a platform that integrates biomedical data, scientific literature, and proprietary algorithms to support target identification and compound optimization. These cases highlight how cross-sector collaboration enables scalable and impactful AI deployment in real-world pharmaceutical settings.

Roadmap for Future Implementation

Building AI-Readiness in Pharmaceutical Organizations

Pharmaceutical organizations need to create AI-ready cultures to access the complete transformative potential that AI brings. Organizations must integrate new technologies into their operations together with transforming workplace culture along with operations. All members of staff need digital education alongside AI training to become ready for strategic leadership roles which lead to innovative goals that produce effective AI adoption results [24]. A robust change management plan is essential to address resistance and ensure a smooth transition from conventional methods to AI-augmented processes.

Institutional Investment in Talent and Infrastructure

Companies need to implement structured AI systems through combined capabilities in data science together with customizable infrastructure models. Pharmaceutical organizations must create ongoing programs to hire and keep professional teams consisting of interdisciplinary members who specialize in bioinformatics together with machine learning and clinical pharmacology. Simultaneously, investments in data lakes, secure cloud platforms, and HPC resources will empower AI tools to function efficiently and securely at scale. Partnerships between pharmaceutical companies and academic institutions alongside AI startups will help meet the talent shortage along with driving new product development [25].

Continuous Evaluation and Innovation Loops

To become future-ready AI implementation must set up ongoing feedback systems and innovate in continuous development cycles. Organizational development is adjusted based on user feedback derived from real-time operational performance data, which informs the interpretation of functional outcomes. Embracing agile methodologies allows teams to respond to new data, regulatory shifts, and emerging scientific insights swiftly. Better drug development requires organizations to build internal systems with ethical benchmarks for measuring AI use which supports both sustainability and corporate responsibility [26].

Conclusion

Summary of Key Strategies and Considerations

The framework combines operational guidelines with ethical principles and regulatory specifications which guide AI drug research activity. AI-driven tools require both data curation and model validation combined with risk mitigation steps during implementation together with interdisciplinary cooperation to retain scientific validity while achieving practical results. By adopting best practices in AI development and deployment, pharmaceutical organizations can streamline discovery pipelines, enhance decision-making, and reduce development costs and timelines [27].

Emphasis on Strategic Partnerships and Innovation Culture

When IT links up with pharmaceutical sectors and when academia teams up with industries and global corporations collaborate with startups strategic alliances become vital. These collaborations are essential for accessing diverse data sources, technological expertise, and regulatory guidance. Equally important is cultivating a culture of innovation within organizations, where cross-functional teams are encouraged to experiment, iterate, and co-develop AI solutions [28]. Building AI-readiness goes beyond infrastructure; it also involves empowering people and processes to adapt and evolve.

Vision for the Future: Toward Precision Pharmacology with AI

Looking ahead, the integration of AI into pharmaceutical research is poised to move the industry closer to precision pharmacology where therapies are tailored not just to diseases, but to individual genetic profiles, environments, and behaviors. AI will serve as a catalyst for this transformation, enabling real-time learning, predictive modeling, and dynamic treatment optimization. With continued investment, ethical oversight, and strategic foresight, AI can unlock the next era of personalized, efficient, and impactful medication development [29].

References

1. Gulshan, V., Peng, L., Coram, M., Stumpe, M. C., Wu, D., Narayanaswamy, A., & Webster, D. R. (2016). Development and validation of a deep learning algorithm for detection of diabetic retinopathy in retinal fundus photographs. *JAMA*, *316*(22), 2402.
2. Kermany, D. S., Goldbaum, M., Cai, W., Valentim, C. C. S., Liang, H., Baxter, S. L., & Zhang, K. (2018). Identifying medical diagnoses and treatable diseases by image-based deep learning. *Cell*, *172*(5), 1122–1131.e9.
3. Esteva, A., Kuprel, B., Novoa, R. A., Ko, J., Swetter, S. M., Blau, H. M., & Thrun, S. (2017). Dermatologist-level classification of skin cancer with deep neural networks. *Nature*, *542*(7639), 115–118.
4. Aminabee, S. K., Prabhakar, M. C., Prasad, R. G. S. V., & Lakshmana Rao, A. (2011). Screening the pharmacological activity of cerium oxide nanoparticles in-vitro. *Biomedical and Pharmacology Journal*, *4*(2), 287–289.
5. Cheng, J. Z., Ni, D., Chou, Y. H., Qin, J., Tiu, C. M., Chang, Y. C., & Chen, C. M. (2016). Computer-aided diagnosis with deep learning architecture: Applications to breast lesions in US images and pulmonary nodules in CT scans. *Scientific Reports*, *6*, 24454.
6. Murdoch, T. B., & Detsky, A. S. (2013). The inevitable application of big data to health care. *JAMA*, *309*(13), 1351–1352.
7. Jiang, F., Jiang, Y., Zhi, H., Dong, Y., Li, H., Ma, S., & Wang, Y. (2017). Artificial intelligence in healthcare: Past, present and future. *Stroke and Vascular Neurology*, *21*, 230–243.

8. Aminabee, S. K., Lakshmana Rao, A., Sowmya, K., Nymisha, D., Kusuma Naga Lakshmi, K., Manikanta, K. V. N. S., & Praveen Kumar, P. (2019). Evaluation of analgesic activity of *Ficus palmata*. *Iranian Journal of Pharmaceutical Sciences*, *15*(3), 47–60.
9. Johnson, K. W., Torres Soto, J., Glicksberg, B. S., Shameer, K., Miotto, R., Ali, M., & Dudley, J. T. (2018). Artificial intelligence in cardiology. *Journal of the American College of Cardiology*, *71*(23), 2668–2679.
10. Tang, A., Tam, R., Cadrin-Chênevert, A., Guest, W., Chong, J., Barfett, J., … &, Canadian Association of Radiologists (2018). Canadian Association of Radiologists white paper on artificial intelligence in radiology. *Canadian Association of Radiologists Journal*, *69*(2), 120–135.
11. De Fauw, J., Ledsam, J. R., Romera-Paredes, B., Nikolov, S., Tomasev, N., Blackwell, S., & Suleyman, M. (2018). Clinically applicable deep learning for diagnosis and referral in retinal disease. *Nature Medicine*, *24*(9), 1342–1350.
12. Aminabee, S. K., Lakshmana Rao, A., & Chinna Eswaraiah, M. (2020). In-vivo antioxidant activity of different fractions of *Indigofera barberi* against paracetamol-induced toxicity in rats. *Turkish Journal of Pharmaceutical Sciences*, *17*(2), 136–140.
13. Slomka, P. J., Dey, D., Berman, D. S., & Germano, G. (2017). Cardiac imaging: Working towards fully-automated machine analysis and interpretation. *Expert Review of Medical Devices*, *14*, 197–212.
14. Prasanth, D. S. N. B. K., Aminabee, S. K., Lakshmana Rao, A., Teja, N., Bhargavi, K., Monika, C., Pujitha, B., Sandhya, T., Lalitha, A., & Siva Prasad, P. (2020). Anthelmintic activity of *Mansoa alliacea* against *Pheretima posthuma*: In-vitro and in-silico approach. *Thai Journal of Pharmaceutical Sciences*, *4*(3), 186–196.
15. Prasanth, D. S. N. B. K., Aminabee, S. K., Lakshmana Rao, A., Guntupalli, C., Reddy, A. R., Kulandaivelu, U., Rao, S. N. K., & Rajeshwari, P. (2021). Inhibitory effects of *Mansoa alliacea* in Freund's adjuvant arthritis on inflammatory markers and its confirmation by in-silico strategy. *Thai Journal of Pharmaceutical Sciences*, *45*(6), 532–544.
16. Cheng, J. Z., Ni, D., Chou, Y. H., Qin, J., Tiu, C. M., Chang, Y. C., & Wang, T. (2016). Computer-aided diagnosis with deep learning architecture: Applications to breast lesions in US images and pulmonary nodules in CT scans. *Scientific Reports*, *6*, 24454.
17. Jiang, F., Jiang, Y., Zhi, H., Dong, Y., Li, H., Ma, S., …, & Wang, Y. (2017). Artificial intelligence in healthcare: Past, present and future. *Stroke and Vascular Neurology*, *2*(4), 230–243.
18. Aminabee, S. K., Santhi Krupa, D., Hanumanth Rao, K., Sirisha, V., Anitha Kumari, V., Nagasen, D., Sujiya, B., & Leelavati, T. S. (2023). Pharmacoeconomic analysis of biologic vs. biosimilar therapies in rheumatoid arthritis. *International Journal of Chemical and Biochemical Sciences*, *24*(4), 395–400.
19. Leelavati, T. S., Madhavi, S., Kamal, G., Raju, P. V. M., Susmitha, K., Vinod, M., & Aminabee, S. K. (2023). Revolutionizing healthcare delivery: Telemedicine's influence on access and patient satisfaction. *International Journal of Chemical and Biochemical Sciences*, *24*(5), 106–115.
20. Slomka, P. J., Betancur, J., Liang, J. X., & Dey, D. (2017). Cardiac imaging: Working towards fully-automated machine analysis and interpretation. *Expert Review of Medical Devices*, *14*(3), 197–212.
21. Lakhani, P., & Sundaram, B. (2017). Deep learning at chest radiography: Automated classification of pulmonary tuberculosis by using convolutional neural networks. *Radiology*, *284*(2), 574–582.
22. Aminabee, S. K., Devi Mallika, K., & Lakshmana Rao, A. (2023). Natural resources in management and treatment of diseases: A review. *Pharma Times*, *55*(11), 7–10.
23. Sitapati, A., Kim, H., Berkovich, B., Marmor, R., Singh, S., El-Kareh, R., …, & Ohno-Machado, L. (2017). Integrated precision medicine: The role of electronic health records in delivering personalized treatment. *Wiley Interdisciplinary Reviews: Systems Biology and Medicine*, *9*(6), e1378.

24. Niu, J., Tang, W., Xu, F., Zhou, X., & Song, Y. (2016). Global research on artificial intelligence from 1990–2014: Spatially-explicit bibliometric analysis. *ISPRS International Journal of Geo-Information*, *5*(5), 66.
25. Aminabee, S. K., & Lakshmana Rao, A. (2024). Computational identification of selected bioactive compounds from *Cedrus deodara* as inhibitors against SARS-CoV-2 main protease: A pharmacoinformatics study. *Indian Drugs*, *61*(2), 78–91.
26. Char, D. S., Shah, N. H., & Magnus, D. (2018). Implementing machine learning in health care-addressing ethical challenges. *New England Journal of Medicine*, *378*(11), 981–983.
27. Ravi Shankar, K., Aminabee, S. K., Ramana, G., Chenchu Lakshmi, K. N. V., & Indusree, G. (2024). Formulation and evaluation of propranolol hydrochloride floating tablets by 32 factorial design. *International Journal of Drug Delivery Technology*, *14*(4), 2060–2067.
28. Fonseca, C. G., Backhaus, M., Bluemke, D. A., Britten, R. D., Chung, J. D., Cowan, B. R., & Young, A. A. (2011). The Cardiac Atlas Project-An imaging database for computational modeling and statistical Atlases of the heart. *Bioinformatics*, *27*(16), 2288–2295.
29. Jimenez-Del-Toro, O., Müller, H., & Kelm, B. M., et al. (2016). Cloud-based evaluation of anatomical structure segmentation and landmark detection algorithms: VISCERAL anatomy benchmarks. *IEEE Transactions on Medical Imaging*, *35*(11), 2459–2475.

Index

Note: page numbers in *italics* refer to figures and **bold** refer to tables.

absorption, distribution, metabolism, excretion, and toxicity (ADMET) 5, 7, 24, 32, 42, 50, 87, 93–95, 103, 141–143, 157–159, **158**; datasets 158–159; pharmacokinetic/pharmacodynamic models 158; predictive modeling for 157–158; *see also* toxicity assessment
academia *vs.* industry 63
accountability 13, 40, 63, 113, 117, 130, 146, 164, 165, 180
active learning 159; *see also* learning
adaptive trial design 143–144, 147, 148
adverse drug reactions (ADRs) 16, 29, 65, 78, 100, 174
agile methodologies 177, 178, 183
algorithmic bias 13, 44, 61, 117, 148, 177; *see also* bias
algorithm library 8
AlphaFold 33, 53, 60, 69, 73, 76, 89, 136, 154, 167, 176
Alzheimer 92, 139
Amazon Web Services (AWS) 56, 177
analysis: big data 23, 60–61, 117, 132, 152; biological dataset 69; data 4, 7, 16, 23, 25, 27, 41, 61, 69, 72, 80, 99, 129, 143, 166, 176, 179; on genetic data 33; histopathological 105–106; multi-omics 40, 69, 107–108, 110; of patent registrations 51; of protein-ligand binding interactions 36; real-world data 41; sentiment 4, 71
Application Programming Interfaces (APIs) 58
Artificial General Intelligence (AGI) 166–167
artificial intelligence (AI) 1, **13**, 48, 99, 153–154; clinical development 99–114, **112**; fundamentals of 2–4, *3*; future of 13–16, 40–43, *42*; global collaborations in *14*, 44; in healthcare *11*; integration of *7*, 34–37, *36*; role of *6*, 43, 135–136; *see also* bioinformatics; case studies; cognitive computing; deep learning (DL); generative AI; machine learning (ML); natural language processing (NLP); robotics system; technology
Artificial neural networks (ANNs) 3, 60
assessment: clinical trial 32, 111; pharmacokinetic and toxicological 93; risk 181–182, **182**; safety 95, 104–106, 109–110
ATAC-seq data 102
atomic resolution 33, 53, 89
AtomNet platform 10, 73, 74, 146
automated closed-loop systems 166
automation 8, 43, 54, 69, 85, 99, 100, 148, 181

Bayesian Networks 4, 8
Bayesian optimization 91, 138, 144
BenevolentAI 10, 65, 136, 145–146, 154, 182–183
best practices 177–178, **179**; for implementation 177–178, **179**
bias 165, 177, 180; algorithmic 13, 44, 61, 117, 148, 177; data 55, 79–80, 86; mitigation 113, 124
Bidirectional Encoder Representations from Transformers for Biomedical Text Mining (BioBERT) 175, 176
big data analytics 23, 60–61, 117, 132, 152
bioactivity data 54, 55, 58; *see also* data
bioavailability 5, 14, 29, 87, 91, 142, 174

bioinformatics 33, 43, 138, 154, 167, 179, 183
biological data 24, 27, 32, 33, 49, 50, 54, 68–70, 82, 94, 112, 154, 155; *see also* data
biomarkers 24, 27, 35, 40, 43, 51–52, 68, 70, 73, 74, 78, 108, 144, 154, 155, 174, 176; *see also* personalized medicine; pharmacogenomics
biomedical datasets 10, 34, 38, 55–56, 65, 145, 148, 175, 177; *see also* datasets
black-box models 14, 79, 86, 97, 146, 164
blockchain technology 34, 35–37, 41, 43, 63, 80, 107, 108; *see also* technology

cancer 4, 32, 74, 75, 92–93, 101–102, 112, 138–139, 144, 167; *see also* oncology
cardiotoxicity 94, 143, 157
case studies 135–150, 182–183; adaptive trial design 143–144; ADME and toxicity 142–143; Atomwise operations 146; BenevolentAI 145–146; biomarker discovery 144; challenges and future perspectives 148–149; CNN model 143; collaborative success stories 182–183; COVID-19 140, 182; data transparency 146; decision-making systems 147; drug repurposing 140–141; generated models 141; hit identification and lead optimization 141–142; industry use 145–146; kinase targets 138–139, *139*; knowledge graph applications 140–141; lead optimization 141–142, *142*; methodological framework 137–138; network pharmacology models 144–145; neurodegenerative disease targets 139; omics and systems biology 144–145; overview 135–136; patient stratification 143; preclinical and clinical trial design 143–144; rare diseases 140–141, 182; and real-world applications 182–183; regulatory and ethical considerations 146–147; in silico evidence 123; target identification 138–139
Central Drugs Standard Control Organization (CDSCO) 119, 180–181
ChEMBL 55, 57, 63, 142
chemical data 49, 50, 54, 59, 63, 103, 154, 160; *see also* data
Chemical Entities of Biological Interest (ChEBI) 58
cheminformatics 52, 54, 61, 94, 154, 176
chromatin immunoprecipitation sequencing (ChIP-seq) 102
clinical data 17, 43, 50–51, 55, 58, 62, 78, 93, 95, 99, 108, 110, 152, 156, 177; *see also* data
clinical development 5, 99–114, **112**; blockchain functions 108; clinical trials 107; DCTs 107; digital twin technology 110–111; drug repurposing 109; IoT 109; long-term drug safety assessment 109–110; multi-omics analysis 107–108; NLP 108–109; personalized medicine 110–112; pharmacovigilance 108–110; post-market surveillance 108–110; regulatory compliance 110–112; SCAs and GANs 107; *see also* preclinical development
clinical trials 32, 39–40, 49, 97, 100, 104, 107, 128–129; assessment 32, 111; data 6, 24, 35, 57, 65, 109, 127, 140, 145; design 5, 29, 43, 99, 143–144, 174; optimization 29, 33–34, 107, 152; *see also* preclinical development
cloud computing platforms 56, **57**
clustering 2, 8, 50, 60–61, 69, 77, 137, 139, 143
cognitive augmentation 166
cognitive computing 2, 176; *see also* artificial intelligence (AI)
collaborative strategies 179–180
communication 63, 117, 118, 129, 179, 181
Compound Identifiers (CIDs) 57
compound screening 16, 152, 160, 172–173; *see also* screening
computational: tools 29–34, 117, 120, 122, **130**, 131, 153
computational model 69, 80, 117, **120**, 120–121, 130–132, 160; BRICS Countries 119; EMA 118; FDA 118; ICH 118–119; predictions 5, 38, 55, 120–121, 159; regulatory bodies and **119**; techniques 118–119, **119**; tools 29–34, **30–31**, 117, 120, 122, **130**, 131, 153
Consolidated Framework for Implementation Research (CFIR) 174
Continuous integration and deployment (CI/CD) 178
convolutional neural networks (CNNs) 3, 27, 73, 94, 101, 136, 143, 146, 157, 175; *see also* deep learning (DL); neural networks
corporate healthcare 17; *see also* healthcare
cost and time efficiency 88

cost reduction 24
COVID-19 pandemic 65, 136, 140, 145, 149, 154, 163, 182
CRISPR gene editing 34, 37, 43, 72
cross-functional teams 178, 184
cross-validation 122, 138, 178
Cryo-Electron Microscopy (Cryo-EM) 53
cutting-edge tools 167; *see also* AlphaFold; tools
cytochrome P450 (CYP) 94

data: analysis 4, 7, 16, 23, 25, 27, 41, 61, 69, 72, 80, 99, 129, 143, 166, 176, 179; bias 55, 79–80, 86; bioactivity 54, 55, 58; biological 24, 27, 32, 33, 49, 50, 54, 68–70, 82, 94, 112, 154, 155; centralization 69, 163; chemical 49, 54, 59, 63, 103, 154, 160; clinical 17, 43, 50–51, 55, 58, 62, 78, 93, 95, 99, 108, 110, 152, 156, 177; curation 137, 177, 183; -driven method 24, 68; EHRs and real-world 99; epigenomic 40, 102; experimental 55–56, 90, 102, 103, 122, 159, 166, 174; FAIR 49, 54, 130–132; genomic 27, 37, 38, 40, 50, 62, 72, 78–80, 101, 112, 125–127, 143; integration 52, 54, 92, 131; IoT 78–79; metabolomic 23, 27, 40, 50; multi-omics 43, 52, 61, 68, 69, 72, 73, 82, 100, 139, 152; preclinical 119–121; privacy 11, 38, 44, 61, 63, 97, 100, 113, 117, 125, 132, 137, 163–164, 168, 175; processing pipelines *59*, 59–61; protection 41, 126–128; quality 6, 14, 49, 120, 148; security 11, 12, **12**, 17, 34, 41, 61–64, *62*, 96, 108, 114, 125, 128, 129, 172, 180; -sharing 41, 54, 56, 63, 80; simulation 120; single-cell transcriptomics 52; sourcing 137; textual 3, 49, 51–52, transcriptomics 94; transparency 146, 177
data collection 52–54; advanced techniques in 52–54; annotated 54–56; ethical and security concerns 61–64; future advancements in 64–65; and management 48–65; overview 48–49; pipelines 59–61; process 49; storage/manage/interoperability 56–59; structural 53; types of 49–52, *51*; *see also* data; datasets
datasets: Bias in biomedical 55–56; biological 68; biomedical 10, 34, 38, 55–56, 65, 145, 148, 175, 177; genetic and molecular 82; and model generalizability 158–159; molecular bioactivity 55; platforms 55; PPI 70; unbiased 48
decentralized clinical trials (DCTs) 99, 107
decision-making systems 147, 164–165
DeepChem 176
DeepDock 73, 74
deep learning (DL) 3, 4, 8, 23, 25, 32, 43, 48, 59–60, 68, **70**, 82, 99, 100–101, 175; application of 42; for neurodegenerative disease targets 139; role of 135–136; *see also* convolutional neural networks (CNNs); neural networks; recurrent neural networks (RNNs)
deep neural network (DNN) 139
deep reinforcement learning (DRL) 102, 104
de novo drug design 81–82, 85, 86–88, 156–157; advantages 88; GANs 86–87; RL 87; VAEs 87
digital clinical trials 128–129; *see also* clinical trials
digital health innovation 131; *see also* innovation
digital innovation 119; *see also* innovation
Digital Object Identifiers (DOIs) 57
digital twin models 42, 43, 105, 110–111, 128, 162
Disease Ontology (DO) 54
documentation 28, 49, 118, 121–122, 125, 128–130, 132, 146, 165, 178
DrugBank 54, 58, 60, 137, 142
drug design 85–97, *87*; ADMET 93–95; challenges in 96–97; de novo 86–88; drug repurposing 92–93; ethical considerations 96–97; federated learning 96; future perspectives 96–97; multi-objective drug optimization 91; and optimization 85–97; overview 85–86; polypharmacology 92–93; quantum computing in 95–96; SBDD 88–90, **90**; virtual screening 94; *see also* drug discovery; molecular docking; toxicity assessment
drug discovery 23–44; applications in 4–6; case studies 9–10; challenges 14–15, 37–40, 96–97; collaborations 15–16; components of *8*; computational tools for 29–34; ethical considerations and societal impact 11–13, 37–40; evolution of 1–2, *153*; opportunities 14–15; overview 23–25; pipelin 6–9;

stages of **174**; transformative change to 25–29; *see also* artificial intelligence (AI); drug design; technology
Drug-Drug Interaction (DDI) 34, 94, 109, 122–123
drug modeling 130
drug repurposing 5, 92–93, *93*, 109, 140–141; approaches 34; automating hypothesis generation 65; COVID-19 pandemic 182; defined 140; NLP systems 29; polypharmacology and 92–93, *93*; transfer learning for 93
drug safety 29, 32, 50, 74, 95, 105, 106, 108–109, 131, 157
drug screening 35; *see also* screening

education 17, 18, 113, 183
electronic health records (EHRs) 24, 38, 48, 50, 60, 61, 65, 69, 78, 79, 99, 108–109, 136, 140, 146, 152, 174, 175
electronic informed consent (eIC) 129
emerging paradigms 166–167
emerging technology 13–14; *see also* Generative AI; technology; transformers
enzymes 1, 32, 73, 75, 94, 138
epigenetic modifications 101–102
epigenomic data 40, 102; *see also* data
epitope prediction 162
ethical considerations 61–64, 96–97, 146–147, 164–165; algorithmic transparency 125; data privacy 125; personalized medicine 126; in silico drug discovery 125–126, *126*; and societal impact 11–13, 37–40; *see also* regulatory considerations
European Medicines Agency (EMA) 38, 44, 71, 80, 86, 95, 97, 100, 111, 118, 119, 123, 124, 128, 129, 146, 165, 178
experimental data 55–56, 90, 102, 103, 122, 159, 166, 174; *see also* data
Explainable AI (XAI) 10, 13, 15, 17, 39, 56, 63, 79, 95, 100, 113, 124, 177–178, 180

federated learning 35–37, 41, 64, 80, 81, 82, 96, 106; data centralization 163; and data privacy 163–164; and decentralized AI frameworks 164; SMPC 164; *see also* learning
feedback loop operational system 159, 178
Findable, Accessible, Interoperable, and Reusable (FAIR) 49, 54, 56, **57**, 130–132; *see also* data
Food and Drug Administration (FDA) 38, 44, 52, 79, 86, 95, 97, 100, 111, 118, 119, 121, 123, 124, 128, 129, 146–148, 165, 178
future trends 152–168; ADMET Prediction 157–159; AlphaFold 154; cheminformatics and bioinformatics 154; in drug target identification 80–82; emerging paradigms 166–167; federated learning and data privacy 163–164; immunogenicity modeling 162–163; lead compound identification and optimization 156–157; overview 152–153; precision medicine 161–162; quantum computing 160; regulatory and ethical considerations 164–165; reinforcement learning and active learning 159; target identification and validation 155–156; tools 153–154; vaccine development 162–163

Gene Ontology (GO) 54
General Data Protection Regulation (GDPR) 62, 64, 80, 81, 96, 108, 114, 125, 127, 137, 163, 180
Generative adversarial networks (GANs) 13, 28, 38, 76, 82, 85, 86, 103, 107, 137, 141, 149, 173, 175
generative AI 13, 17, 25, 28, 80, 82, 103, 141; *see also* artificial intelligence (AI); de novo drug design
genetic algorithms 4, 8, 60
genomics 60, 68, 72, 86, 100, 105, 108, 125, 126, 137, 138, 152, 155, 172, 174; *see also* proteomics
global collaborations *14*, 56, 168
Good Clinical Practice (GCP) 108, 124
Good Laboratory Practice (GLP) 124
Good Machine Learning Practice (GMLP) 39, 147
good manufacturing practices (GMP) 121–122, 124, 132, 147; computational model 121; documentation and reporting requirements 121; VVUQ 122
Google Cloud Platform (GCP) 56
Gradient Boosting Machines (GBMs) 137
graph convolutional networks (GCNs) 103, 139
Graphics Processing Units (GPUs) 56
graph neural networks (GNNs) 34, 60, 70, **71**, 88–89, 100, 101, 137, 140, 156
guide RNA (gRNA) 37

GWAS technology 72, 139; *see also* technology
GxP compliance 124–125

healthcare *78*; AI applications in *11*, *78*; corporate 17; digital twins 43; ethical problems in 117
Health Insurance Portability and Accountability Act (HIPAA) 62, 64, 80, 81, 96, 114, 125, 127, 137, 180
hepatotoxicity 94, 142, 157
high-dimensional chemical space 160
high-performance computing (HPC) 56, 177, 183
high-throughput screening (HTS) 25, 29, 33, 48, 52, 60, 63, 68, 76–77, 135, 141, 148, 172
histopathological analysis 105–106; *see also* analysis
hit identification 77, 85, 103, 141–142, 146
human-AI collaboration 44, 166
Human Genome Project 135
human intelligence 44, 148
hybrid quantum-classical models 95–96, 160
hypothesis generation 58, 64, 65, 71, 82, 145–146

IBM Watson 65, 176, 182
immunogenicity modeling 162–163; epitope prediction and 162; surveillance systems 163; vaccine design 163
implementation 171–184; applications and strategies for 171–184; best practices for 177–178, **179**; continuous evaluation and innovation loops 183; future 183; institutional investment 183; pharmaceutical organizations 183; science for AI adoption 174–175; *see also* medication research
incremental development 178
induced pluripotent stem cells (iPSCs) 53
industry 9, 13, 57, 61, 63–64, 86, 111, 118, 127, 135, 145–146, 167–168, 184
innovation 80; balancing 132; digital 119, 131; loops 183; *see also* technology
in silico evidence 119, 122–123, *123*, 125–126; case studies 123; IND/NDA 122; PBPK and QSP models 122–123
insilico medicine 9, *9*, 136
in silico toxicology 29, 32, 94
institutional investment 183
intellectual property (IP) 52, 63, 126–128; AI-generated discoveries 126–127; data sharing 127–128; patent regulations 126–127
International Chemical Identifier (InChI) 54
International Council for Harmonisation (ICH) 38, 44, 118–119
Internet of Things (IoT) 77, 78–79, 109
interoperability 49, 54, 56–58, **59**, 130, 181
Investigational New Drug (IND) 122

joint ventures 179–180

kinase targets 138–139, *139*
k-nearest neighbors (KNN) 56
Kyoto Encyclopedia of Genes and Genomes (KEGG) 58

lead compound identification: CNNs 157; de novo molecule design 156–157; and optimization 156–157; QSAR modeling 157
lead discovery 4–5, 7, 159
lead optimization 5, 52, 53, 61, 77, 85, 87, 91, 96, 102–106, *104*, 114, 141–142, *142*, 154; *see also* optimization
learning: active 159; federated 35–37, 41, 64, 80–82, 96, 106, 163–164; processes 8; techniques 55, 69, 103, 113, 159; transfer 38, 93, 137, 157; unsupervised 2, 27, 41, 59, 60, 69, 139
literature mining 28, 51, 57, 69, 140, 176
Local Interpretable Model-Agnostic Explanation (LIME) 63, 79, 146, 178
long-term drug safety assessment 109–110; *see also* assessment

machine learning (ML) 2, 4, 23, 25, 38, 43, 48, 59–60, 68, **70**, 99, 175; adaptive trial design optimization 143–144; AI-based predictions 124; application of 24; explainability and bias mitigation 124; GxP compliance 124–125; for high-dimensional chemical space 160; in regulatory considerations 124–125; role of 135–136; *see also* Quantum Machine Learning (QML); reinforcement learning (RL); supervised learning; unsupervised learning
Medical Subject Headings (MeSH) 54
medication research 171–184; Agile methodologies 178; best practices 177–178, **179**; building

interdisciplinary teams 179; case studies 182–183; collaborative strategies 179–180; communication and workflow alignment 179; data curation and quality control 177; drug discovery 172–174; ethical/legal/regulatory considerations 180, **181**; framework for AI integration in 172–175; objectives 172, *173*; overview 171–172; PPPs 179–180; practical frameworks and actionable strategies 171; risk assessment and mitigation 181–182, **182**; technological infrastructure and tools 175–177; transformative role in 171; validation and reproducibility 178; XAI 177–178; *see also* implementation
metabolomics 23, 27, 40, 50, 73–74
microphysiological systems (MPS) 99, 105
mitigation 108, 113, 124, 165, 181–183, **182**
model generalizability 81, 157–159
Model Informed Drug Development (MIDD) 118, 121
molecular bioactivity datasets 55; *see also* datasets
molecular docking 32, 76, 88, *89*, 95, 103–104, 119–120, 146
molecular dynamics (MD) 35, 120
molecular generation 136
molecular modeling techniques 32, 35, 36, 75, 95, 113, 117, 132; *see also* techniques
molecular simulations 35, 36, 64–65, 81, 86, 95, 99, 100, 103, 120, 160
multi-objective drug optimization 91, **92**, 159; Bayesian optimization 91; MPO 91; Pareto front 91
multi-omics data 43, 52, 61, 68, 69, 72, 73, 82, 100, 139, 152; *see also* data
Multi-Parameter Optimization (MPO) 91
multiple imputation by chained equations (MICE) 56

named entity recognition (NER) 3, 54, 176
nanotechnology 149
National Medical Products Administration (NMPA) 119
natural language processing (NLP) 3, 8, 23, 25, 28, 29, 43, 48, 52, 65, 69, 71, **71**, 78, 99, 108–109, 111, 136, 145, 152, 154, 174, 175; drug repurposing 29; for EHRs 108–109, 175; role of 135–136; for target discovery 71; techniques 48, 69, 71; *see also* sentiment analysis; text mining
network pharmacology models 76, 92–93, 144–145
neural networks 79, 86–87, 91, 94, 103, 113, 136, 143, 144, 152, 153, 158; *see also* convolutional neural networks (CNNs); deep learning (DL); recurrent neural networks (RNNs)
neurodegenerative disorders 16, 32, 42, 74, 92, 101, 139, 161
New Drug Applications (NDA) 122
next-generation drug discovery *77*, 113–114
Next-generation sequencing (NGS) 152
Novartis 182–183
novel disease pathways 155
novel drug-binding sites 90

OECD principles 121
omics-based toxicology 105–106
omics-driven target discovery *72*, 72–74
oncology 74, 75, 111, 123, 139, 182; *see also* cancer
ontologies 54, 56–59, **58**, 65, 177
open science *vs.* proprietary tools 129–131, **130**
operational risk 181
optimization 85–97; clinical trial 29, 33–34, 107, 152; compound screening and 172; lead 141–142; and lead compound identification 156–157; MPO 91; multi-objective drug 91, **92**, 159; techniques 87, 138 (*see also* techniques); *see also* drug design
orchestration 8
organ-on-a-chip technologies 99; *see also* technology

Pareto front-based AI models 91
Parkinson's diseases 139
patient-derived models 53–54
patient-derived xenografts (PDXs) 53
patient selection 34, 39, 99, 107; *see also* clinical trial
patient stratification 33, 51, 99, 107–108, 143, 147, 148, 149, 161
PBPK models 118, 122–123
personalized medicine 39–40, 88, 110–112; and clinical trials 39–40; digital twin technology 110–111; FDA/EMA/PMDA 111;

pharmacogenomics for 111–112; quantum computing 111; *see also* biomarkers
personally identifiable information (PII) 38
Pfizer 182–183
pharmaceutical organizations 8–9, 15, 23, 91, 174, 179, 182–184; *see also* medication research
pharmaceutical research 2, 8, 10, 15, 23, 25, 34, 37, 44, 54, 96–97, 117, 146, 163, 184
Pharmaceuticals and Medical Devices Agency (PMDA) 111, 118
pharmacodynamic models 86, 91, 96, 102, 154, 158
pharmacogenomics 111–112; *see also* biomarkers
pharmacokinetics (PK) 27, 32, 43, 50, 55, 58, 60, 77, 89, 91, 96, 102, 109, 137, 153, 157, 158, 175
pharmacovigilance 100, 108–110, 174
phenotypic screening 33; *see also* screening
policymakers 167–168
polypharmacology 92–93, *93*; and drug repurposing 92–93, *93*; and multi-target drug design 74–75; network pharmacology 92–93; patient stratification and 161; target affinity prediction models 92
PopPK modeling 118
populations 12, 38, 62, 64, 105, 110, 111, 113, 122, 124, 131, 139, 180
post-market surveillance 108–110, *110*, 174
precision medicine *145*, 148–149, 161–162; digital twins 162; patient-specific therapies 161; personalized and **162**; targeted therapeutic medicine 161
preclinical data 119–121; computational models **120**, 120–121; QSAR 119–120; virtual screening and simulation data 120; *see also* data
preclinical development 5, 99–114, **106**; ADMET 103; bias mitigation strategies 113; challenges and perspectives 113–114; digital twin technology 105; DRL 104; epigenetic modifications 101–102; federated learning 106; GANs 103; GNNs 101; histopathological analysis 105–106; lead optimization 102; molecular docking 103–104; MPS 105; omics-based toxicology 105–106; overview 99–100; privacy-preserving 114; quantum computing 113–114; safety assessment 104–106; scRNA-seq 101; target identification 100; XAI 113; *see also* clinical development; clinical trials
preclinical trials 128, 143–144; *see also* clinical trials
predictive models 16, 24, 27, 32–34, 68, 77, 78, 99, 110, 137, 157, 163, 167, 174, 179, 184
Principal Component Analysis (PCA) 60, 61, 77
privacy-preserving techniques 62, 81, 114, 168; *see also* techniques
protein-protein interactions (PPIs) 70, 104
proteomics 27, 40, 52, 60, 73, 86, 100, 105, 108, 112, 137, 152, 155, 172; *see also* genomics
PubChem 54, 55, 57, 58, 60, 63, 94, 137
Public-Private Partnerships (PPPs) 15, 17, 179–180

quality control 6, 25, 177
Quantitative Structure-Activity Relationship (QSAR) 94, 119–121, 143, 154, 157
quantitative systems pharmacology (QSP) 118, 122–123
quantum-AI hybrid models 35, 36, 113–114
quantum algorithms 36, 65, 95, 114
quantum chemistry 96, 176
quantum computing 14, 17, 35, 64–65, 80, 81, 86, 95–96, 111, 113–114, 132, 160, *161*; high-dimensional chemical space 160; Hybrid AI-quantum models 95–96, QML 95; quantum chemistry 96; *see also* emerging technology
quantum machine learning (QML) 35, 36, 65, 95, 160; *see also* machine learning

Random Forest (RF) 60
rapid exploration of chemical space 88
rare diseases 16, 38, 55, 107, 140–141, 159, 182
Reach, Effectiveness, Adoption, Implementation, and Maintenance (RE-AIM) 174
readiness spectrum **128**
real-world applications 97, 182–183
Real-World Data (RWD) 41, 52–54, 77–79
real-world evidence (RWE) 51, 65, 77, 131

recurrent neural networks (RNNs) 3, 27, 94, 101, 136, 175; *see also* deep learning (DL); neural networks
regulatory compliance 10, 37, 39, 44, 61, 79, 80, 96, 97, 108, 110–112, 117, 118, 163, 165, 174, 177–178
regulatory considerations 117–132, 146–147, 164–165, **181**; AI/big data/quantum computing 132; bias/reproducibility/accountability 165, 180; CDSCO 180–181; clinical trials 128–129; computational models 118–119, **119**, **120**, 120–121; data protection 126–128; decision-making processes 164–165; digital clinical trials and virtual patients 128–129; digital health innovation 131; of digital twin models 128; EMA 118, 165, 180–181; and ethical implications 117–132; FAIR data 130–131; FDA 118, 165, 180–181; GMP 121–122; HIPAA data 180; ICH 118–119; IP 126–128; ML in 124–125; molecular docking 119–120; open science *vs.* proprietary tools 129–131, **130**; overview 117–118; preclinical data 119–121; readiness spectrum **128**; risk communication 129; RWE 131; in silico evidence 122–123, 125–126; transparency *vs.* commercial interests 130; virtual screening and simulation data 120; *see also* ethical considerations
regulatory evaluation, components of 147
reinforcement learning (RL) 2, 25, 27, 41, 85–87, 91, 141, *142*, 145, 154; active learning 159; for drug optimization 29; feedback loop operational system 159; for multi-objective optimization 159; *see also* machine learning (ML)
remote monitoring 99, 107, 129
reproducibility 49, 56, 118, 120, 124, 129, 130, 158, 165, 178, 180
responsible AI 12–13, **13**, 61, 97
risk assessment: and mitigation 181–182, **182**; operational 181; technical 181
RNA sequencing (RNA-seq) 4
robotics system 2, 166; *see also* artificial intelligence (AI); technology
RoseTTAFold 33

safety assessment 95, 104–106, 109–110; *see also* assessment
screening: compound 16, 152, 160, 172–173; drug 35; phenotypic 33; virtual 24, 28, 32, 53, 75–77, 90, 94, 120, 146, 172
Secure Multi-Party Computation (SMPC) 164
sentiment analysis 4, 71; *see also* analysis; natural language processing (NLP)
Shapley Additive Explanations (SHAP) 63, 79, 113, 146, 178
Simplified Molecular Input Line Entry System (SMILES) 54, 141
simulation data 120; *see also* data
Single-cell RNA sequencing (scRNA-seq) 52–53, 100, 101, 139
skills 18, 27, 167
social media 4, 100, 108, 163
societal impact 11–13, 37–40
software 17, 44, 74–75, 120, 121, 124, 129, 138, 147–148, 160, 165, 175, 176, 178, 180
Software as a Medical Device (SaMD) 124, 165, 180
stakeholders 15, 117, 121, 127, 147
Standard operating procedures (SOPs) 172
structural biology 29, 33, 43, 52, 53, 60, 73, 74
structure-activity relationship (SAR) 23, 52, 102, 173
Structure-Based Drug Design (SBDD) 88–90, **90**; advantages 90; AlphaFold 89; GNNs 88–89; molecular docking 88
supervised learning 2, 27, 55, 59, 60, 69, 102–104, 137; *see also* machine learning (ML)
support vector machines (SVMs) 60, 136, 142
surveillance systems 110, 163
synthetic control arms (SCAs) 99, 107

target affinity prediction 87, 92–93
target flexibility 90
target identification 4, 68–82, 100, *102*, 138–139, 172; challenges 79–80; computational approaches for 69–71; data bias 79–80; de novo 81–82; EHR system 78; federated learning 81; future trends in 80–82; genomic data 72; GNNs 70, **71**, 156; HTS 76–77; IoT data 78–79; metabolomics 73–74; mining genomics/proteomics/transcriptomics data 155; ML and DL technologies 69–70, **70**; molecular docking 75–76; multi-omics data 72–74; NLP 70, **71**; novel disease pathways and biomarkers 155; overview 68–69; pharmacology 74–75; proteomics 73; regulatory and

ethical considerations 79, 80; RWD 77–79; and validation 155–156; virtual screening 75–77
target selection 1, 8, 24, 25, 68, 70, 72
target validation 53, 70, 75–77, 172
t-Distributed Stochastic Neighbor Embedding (t-SNE) 60, 61
technical risks 181
techniques: computational 118–119, **119**; in data collection 52–54; drug screening 35; learning 55, 69, 103, 113, 159; MD 35; molecular modeling 32, 35, 36, 75, 95, 113, 117, 132; NLP 48, 69, 71; optimization 87, 138; privacy-preserving 62, 81, 114, 168; SHAP and LIME 146; VVUQ 122; XAI 10; *see also* tools
technological infrastructure: AI models in practice 175; HPC 177; platforms and software 176, *176*; and tools 175–177
technology **26**; ACI 34; blockchain 34, 35–37, 41, 43, 63, 80, 107, 108; CRISPR gene editing 34, 37, 43, 72; digital twin 105; emerging 13–14; GWAS 72, 139; NLP 3; organ-on-a-chip 99; *see also* artificial intelligence (AI); innovation; robotics system; tools
Tensor Processing Units (TPUs) 56
text mining 3, 71, 175; *see also* natural language processing (NLP)
textual data 3, 49, 51–52; *see also* data
three-dimensional (3D) 50, 53, 89, 105, 154
tools: computational 29–34, **30–31**, 117, 120, 122, **130**, 131, 153; cutting-edge 167; open-source 129–130; structural biology 33; and technological infrastructure 175–177; *see also* techniques
toxicity assessment 93–95, 142–143; ADMET prediction and 94; DDI 94; future directions 95; hepatotoxicity 94; virtual screening 94; XAI techniques 95
training approaches 137
transcriptomics 27, 40, 50, 52–53, 68, 75, 92, 100, 112, 137, 154–155, 172
transfer learning 38, 93, 137, 157; *see also* learning
transformers 13, 28, 136, 141, 175; *see also* emerging technology
transparency *vs.* commercial interests 130

Uniform Manifold Approximation and Projection (UMAP) 60, 61
unsupervised learning 2, 27, 41, 59, 60, 69, 139; *see also* learning; machine learning (ML)

vaccine development 162–163
validation 53, 75, 119, **120**, 122, 138, 155–156, 165, 172, 178; *see also* target identification
variational autoencoders (VAEs) 28, 38, 76, 85, 86, 87, 103, 141, 156, 173, 175; *see also* deep learning (DL); machine learning (ML)
verification, validation, and uncertainty quantification (VVUQ) 122
virtual bioequivalence 123; *see also* computational model
virtual environments 125, 129
virtual patients 128–129, 131
virtual screening 24, 28, 32, 53, 75–77, 90, 94, 120, 146, 172; *see also* screening

Made in the USA
Las Vegas, NV
19 September 2026

b9cab86a-27ef-433a-8ce9-4edc8f106784R02